Contents

> *"I dedicate this book to all who read it with oot fallin asleep"*

Building ships to building teams

Introduction

I started this book twenty years ago when I was working in the local authority and called it "Around the block and back again". Twenty years on and I am a little bit wiser and more experienced having spent the last fifteen years working in the NHS.

I realised when reflecting on what to write that it was important to include my whole working career as what I learnt in the very early days has stood me in good stead for what I do now. It was also important to recognise my working-class background and the values which were instilled in me from my wonderful parents. Respect and social justice were two of the most important aspects of that learning.

I have also included some important life changes in the process of travelling through my working life. Marriage, death, fatherhood, sickness, education attainment and many other highs and bumps along the road which have helped me to create a clear perspective of work and life balance. This book is not supposed to be a literal work of art but more a reflection and celebration of my life and the people I have had the pleasure of working with and in some cases, those who I haven't.

I hope to explore the cultural variations in the different organisations I have worked for and the values and principals they have operated under. The autocratic and the engagers, the rebels and reformists, the politics and the power trips the deceit and the delight, the bullshit and the rhetoric, the passionate and the innovators, the creative and the bureaucrats, the shirkers and the workers, the compassionate and the bullies, the front line staff and the management, the theorists and the pragmatists, the doers and the do nothings, the jokers and the jesters, the leaders and the followers, the wingers and the moaners, the inspirers and the inspired, and the reason we

BUILDING SHIPS
TO BUILDING
TEAMS

W A L L Y   C H A R L T O N

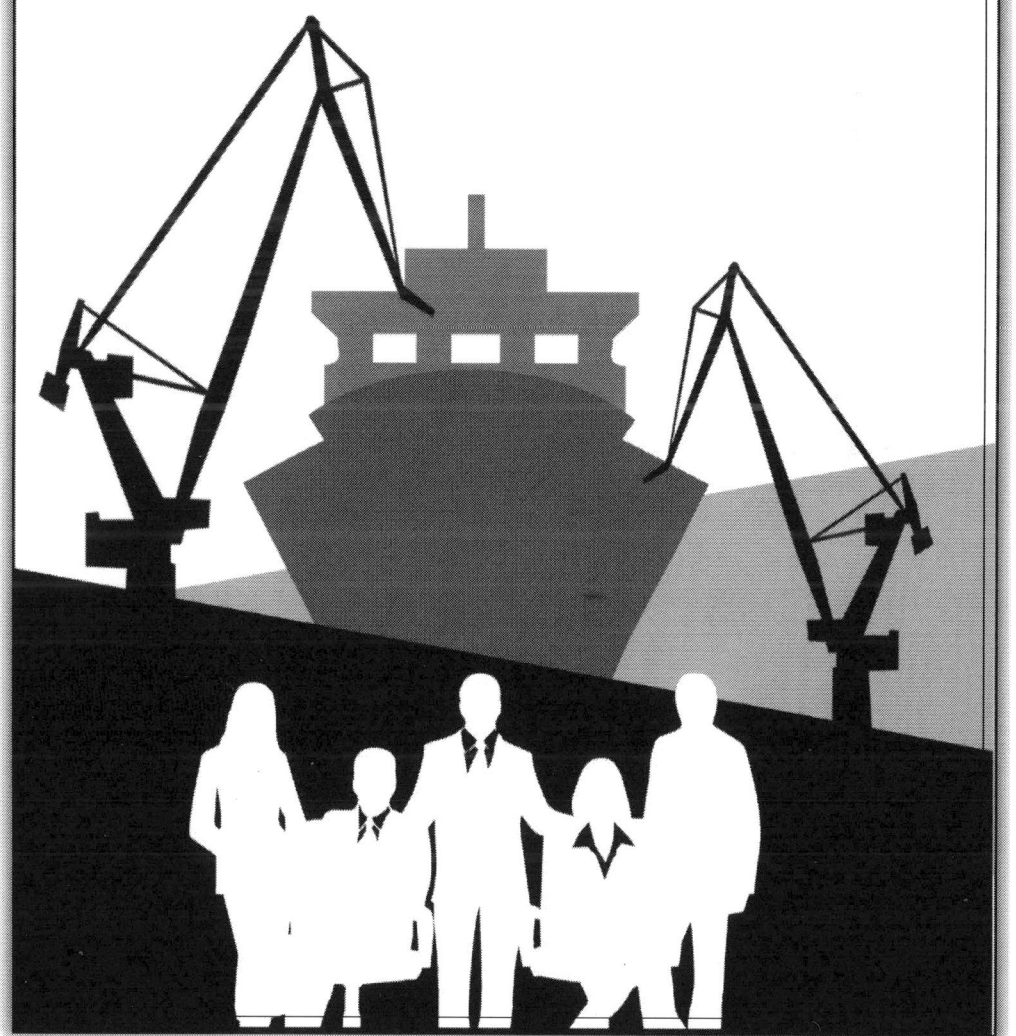

To Eleanor Rose, my beautiful granddaughter who has made mine and Debbie's heart melt with love

Your laugh, your smile your funny face
Your beautiful blonde hair which flows like lace
Your squeals and shouts, your funny little walk
I can't wait for the day when you talk
And say Grandad

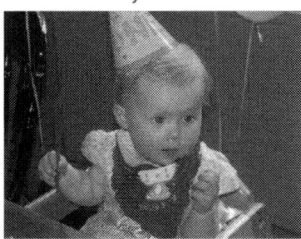

all work for the public sector but often fail to put them central to everything we do, the patients and the public.

Over the coming chapters I will explore the above in more detail and hopefully shed some light on why people act in the way they do with one or two stories of my working life. I will also provide some basic tools and techniques on how to overcome some of the many micro and macro challenges we all must deal with.

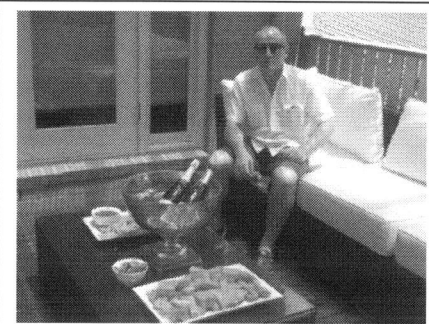
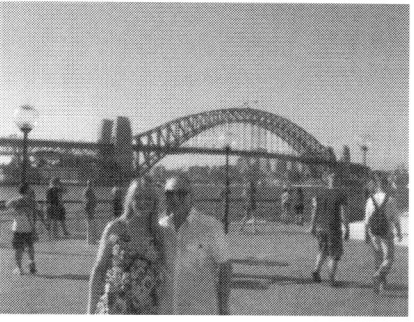
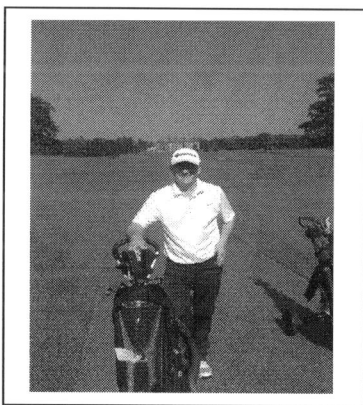

Engage, Empower , Sustain. My principals of working life.

This is me

Born within sight of the River Tyne (this makes me a real Geordie) on the 20th April 1963. I was the youngest of four children with two older brothers and one older sister. My sister Bev and brothers Malc and Will who I am close to now as I was when we all squeezed into the houses we lived in at Gaynor's Terrace, Rosehill Terrace, Martin Road and finally Kent Avenue.

My dad, Walter, served his time down the ship yards as a welder and was the most caring, compassionate and ethical man who will ever walk this earth. He was a gentleman who instilled trust, loyalty and calmness within me. He was a character and a hardworking man who loved his family and a sing a long and also a couple of pints and a whisky and he was one hell of a footballer. I can honestly say I can't remember my dad losing his temper.

My mam, Gladys was an unbelievably hard-working individual who give us everything we wanted even though I know her, and dad went without. She was super confident and did not have a problem standing up to anyone regardless of who they were. She also hated bullies, or any form of injustice and she would challenge anybody openly if she seen this happen. She was always up for a challenge and a good laugh and she also loved her family parties and sing along. I had a wonderful loving and safe childhood where I learnt so much from my family and I strongly believe those principals my mam and dad followed are engrained in the person I am today. They have sadly passed but I Loved them both dearly and they have left me and my family with nothing but happy memories. There isn't a day that goes by without me using a touch of their principals.

Thank you to my two wonderful sons Craig and Liam and my beautiful daughter in law Ashleigh and my future daughter in law Lucy for giving me the kick to write this meandering tale of my working life. They have all been brought up in a working-class area on a council estate and rode all the challenges which come with that. They have made us all proud.

I dedicate this book to Debbie, my wonderful wife who has the patience of a saint and a heart as big as the Tyne Bridge. I will be forever in your debt as I owe you so much. Love, you xxxxx

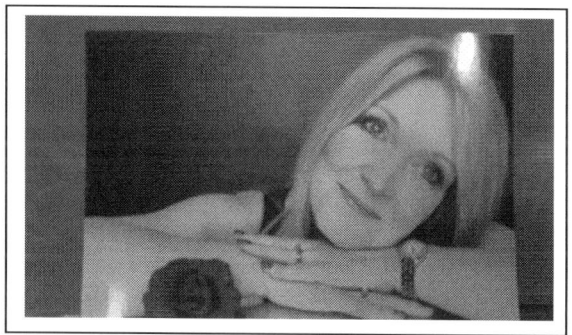

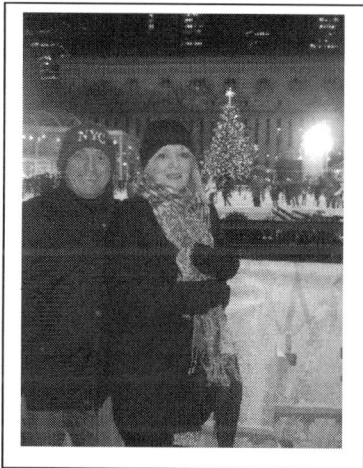

"Don't dream about it strive to become it. We can all be whatever we want to be, you just need to work at it and remember it's the journey not the arrival which is the most rewarding "

Chapter 1

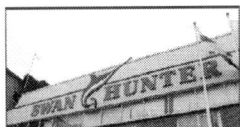

Doon the Yards

I have had the good fortune of working with many people with various characteristics and my first experience of this was meeting a guy called Tommy Moss (my journeyman, mentor and body guard). A proper hard man but I will come back to Tommy later in this chapter.

20th August 1979 – I awoke to the sound of something that I would despise for the rest of my working days, the bloody alarm clock and in 1979 it was a big old wind up contraption which had bells on it like St Pauls Cathedral. My first day at work, I was shitting myself. My dad was telling me everything will be fine whilst my two brothers were filling me in with all kinds of stories which had me petrified. Watch oot for this and divvunt dey that or the blokes will throw you in the Tyne. The scary bit for me was catching the bus with all the other shipyard workers with my spanking brand-new navy blue boiler suit.

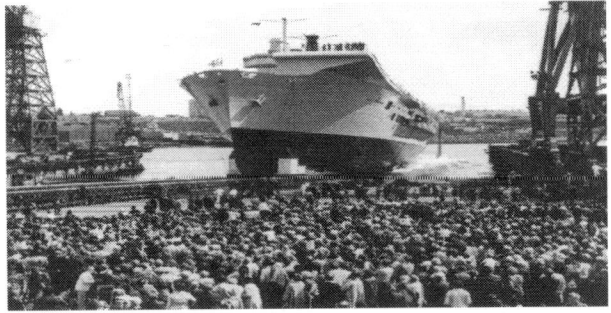

The launch of HMS Ark Royal 1981 at Swan Hunter yard, Wallsend – I was one of many Shipwrights who helped launch the ship.

The bus took me from Howdon to Wallsend (the No 322 or 323) then I jumped on another one (the No 44/45) which dropped me outside of the Swan Hunter training centre which was situated behind the Neptune yard and Wallsend Dry dock where my Dad and both my brothers worked at some point in the 60s, 70s and 80s. I will never forget that bus journey.

When the doors opened for me to enter the bus, a bloody cloud of smoke bellowed out from the bus, I thought the thing was on fire. It didn't improve when I got on the bus, I could hardly see people for the fag smoke and the smell of rollies and No6 fags was overwhelming, and I was a smoker!!!, but I had never experienced anything like that in my life. It is a memory I often think about when I am listening to any debates re the no smoking campaigns today, if they think it was bad putting up with smokers in a bar or the bookies try walking onto a bus filled with blokes and a few women smoking like hell, you were anti-social if you didn't smoke, wow how things have changed for the better.

My life down the shipyards was an experience that has stayed with me, and something I am proud to refer to today when I am presenting lectures or training. I learnt about hierarchy and I can assure you that apprentices were at the bottom of the ladder and you had to earn any form of respect. There were guys who had worked there all their lives and you did not cross them, if you did then expect a hard kick up the arse. You did what you were told from your tradesman who was a modern-day mentor but without governance. Cross him at your peril.

My first year working for Swan Hunter was spent at the training centre on Warwick road in Walker and Newcastle College where I was taught the theory of engineering and also learnt how to bet, drink, smoke and appreciate real friendship and camaraderie as over those first twelve months I developed really strong bonds with the other apprentices within my group, we were all shipwrights and proud of it, I think, or was it that we were all shipwrights because wu fatha had got us the job or there were nee other jobs

9

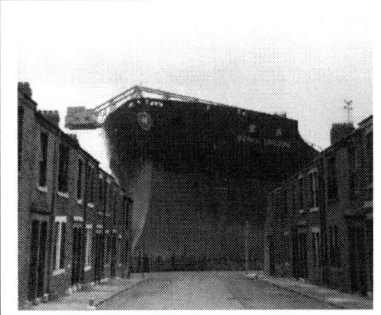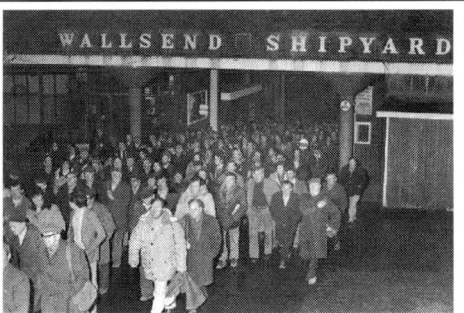

available. I'm not too sure which category I sat in, but one thing is for certain, nearly forty years on I can say that I was proud to be a shipbuilder. The yards were not only where I served my time, but they were my heritage, my roots and where you learnt about the proud history of the skilled people who worked there. Wallsend has a history which is built on shipbuilding and mining and it is critical that we never forget that.

College was not my first experience of hierarchy; after all, I did attend school on most days!! But it was the first time I had experienced the difference from school and the reality of working life. We had three lecturers that were all different:

I will not mention their names, but I will never forget them as each one left there negative and positive marks on me which in a perverse way helped me prepare myself for meeting the real shipyard workforce.

- Lecturer one reminded me of most of my teachers, a know all who had little respect for us first year apprentices and who tried to rule with authority but was actually, a decent guy.
- Lecturer two was an "I want to be everybody's mate" type of bloke as long as you don't cross me, which unfortunately I did.

- Lecturer three was the most laid-back bloke in the world, he didn't like any fuss, and he just wanted to show you how to build things, especially fabricated horses and riders for some bizarre reason. He was unbelievably intelligent and always give me the impression of a sixties hippy, he often spoke of the marches and concerts he attended.

The point I am trying to make is these three guys were completely different. They dressed and presented completely different but they all taught me something. All three showed principals ranging from autocracy to impartial engagement. What I didn't realise at the time that all three of their traits would help me to understand the complexity of people, teams and organisations.

I had "run ins" with two, guess which ones. Yep, lecturer one and two.

Our first classroom session was with lecturer one and he was giving us an overview of the course and the dos and don'ts. Most of the guys in my group had switched off after ten minutes as his dulcet negative tones were boring us rigid, telling us we were now in the adult world and that we would be treat like adults. I never heard anything positive, seriously it was all negative. If you're late we will bollick you, if your early we will make you wait outside the classroom, speak when your spoken to yada yada yada and then the straw that broke the camel's back, "address me as sir or Mr.......". I pitched up, and was then bollicked for not raising my hand. For fucks sake, I thought I had finished school and I was in the big bad world, obviously not. Anyway, I finally asked the question "excuse me sir will you please address me as Mr Charlton". Weheeeyyyy, the man went red with anger. I was not being arsey or difficult I just felt that I was being treated like a piece of dirt, so I repeated myself. "I am more than happy to call you sir or Mr .... But can you please do the same for me or I am more than happy to be called Wally if you want to be called by your first name". The classroom was silent, and I thought he was going to explode, but he didn't he actually started to laugh and then introduced himself using his first name. From that moment on I realised that challenging someone in a positive way when you feel passionate about something is worth doing. I have a huge amount of respect for lecturer one and to this day I remember the line he told us to use when we want to impress people. "Don't tell them you're a ship yard worker tell them you're a ship construction engineer" what a great guy.

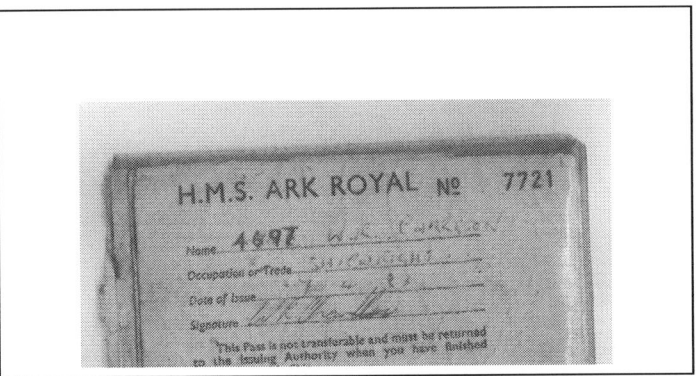

There is no doubt that I am not a saint and I like a good laugh and joke, especially at work. After all we spend a large proportion of our time there and this doesn't mean that I don't work hard it just helps me be the person I am. This trait has been with me since I can remember, and it is definitely something which I learnt from my mother and father and my brothers and sister.

Lecturer two was a similar type of guy until the day I disagreed with him. I can't remember what the debate was about, but I was not agreeing with what he was saying which he didn't take kindly to. He asked me to leave the classroom, and stand outside, back to school again.

"If your glass is always half empty then you have a hard road ahead of you"

I did not want to continue with the debate as I could see he was very angry, so I stepped outside just like he said.

The tossa followed me outside and proceeded to escort me up some stairs which led to his office. This was an old-school building and the stairs were only wide enough for one person to walk up. He then proceeded to grab my neck from behind and he pinned me to the wall. "If you ever cross me again I will fuckin make your life hell both here and back at the training centre". I can honestly say I was gobsmacked and couldn't say anything, so I grabbed the lapels of his jacket pushed him to one side and started to make my way back down the stairs. What was even more surprising was my fellow Shipwrights were heading up the stairs as they knew something was wrong; believe me I was really pleased to see them as I thought this bloke was going to kick the shite out of me. I told them there was nowt a matter and walked back into the classroom with them. We were closely followed by lecturer two who continued with the lesson as if nothing had happened.

The Lesson I learnt was you need to know when to back off and know when to stay in the debate. Agree to disagree unless you have solid evidence that says otherwise and even then, some people will always be right even when they are wrong, but you must learn when to pick your battles and when to withdraw with dignity and, never trust a bloke with a Tweed jacket.

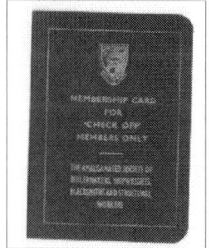 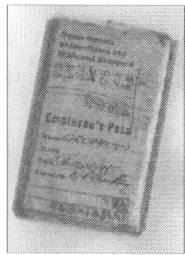

"Never be frightened to fight your corner but always know when to retreat"

I can't finish this chapter without mentioning some of the tutors who give us some great advice and who we learnt so much from during my first twelve months at Swan Hunters and some of the great friendships which evolved during that period and continue to this day. To Eddie Barass, Roy Murphy. Mark (Blacky) Blacklock, Tony, Foz, Mal McVeigh, Fudgie and all the other guys, thanks for the piss takes and comradeship.

Tom Shipley, my training school supervisor looked older than tea with a breadth of knowledge which I only dreamed of. He was old school, dressed in a smart suite, shirt and tie with a pipe which seemed glued to his mouth. A man of small stature but he commanded a room when he walked into it. A leader of young men and respected by all, he had been there and done it, built many ships and led teams of rough arse, hardnosed shipyard workers with dignity and respect.

Bill Shaftoe was our burning instructor, yes he taught us to burn metal using oxy and acetylene gas. I remember one afternoon; we were all situated in our burning bays with benches in front of us, six lads one side and six the other, facing each other. One of my mates, Fossy turned to me and said, "can you smell gas" I had a quick sniff and said "I, a can". By this time some of the other lads, Blacky, big Mal, Roy and Tony were all sniffing the air like a bunch of mere cats. They started to let Billy know there was a smell of gas. Billy came over to our bays and told us to turn everything off, he then turned to the lads on the other side of the work shop (approximately ten feet away) and just as he told them to turn their gas of Eddy Barrass lit his flame with the igniter and a huge flame shot across the work shop about twenty feet, we all dived under the benches, but it was too late for Billy, he caught it full in the face and was burnt pretty badly. It was a wakeup call to what we would face down the yards and how dangerous the yards were. This was no playground it was a very dangerous place and as if we didn't know beforehand we certainly knew now and we were still in the training centre!!!

September 23, 1976 3 years before I started at Swan Hunter Shipbuilders, HMS Glasgow was being built in the Neptune Yard and on that September morning it took the lives of eight men. It is thought the fire at Swan Hunter's Neptune yard was started by a welder's torch after gas had been leaking from an oxygen cylinder. Six other shipyard workers were also injured. We were not in the school yard now we were in an environment that was dangerous and harsh where safety was critical and this dreadful and fatal accident was proof. Billy was off work for a number of weeks and never really recovered from that accident, but it did learn me a lesson of when to focus and when to relax and have a bit "crack and daft carry on" at work.

Happier memories of my first year were the games of football at bait time with the "joiners" on the all-weather (all weather my arse) sand and stone pitch at the back of the training centre. We all played with our safety boots on (steel toe caps) and it was anything but friendly. Pride for your trade was at stake and these games were played with passion, skill and a boat load (pardon the pun) of blood and guts. Some of these guys I played with, and against, later became my team mates when we represented Swan Hunter football team and what a team we were– happy days indeed.

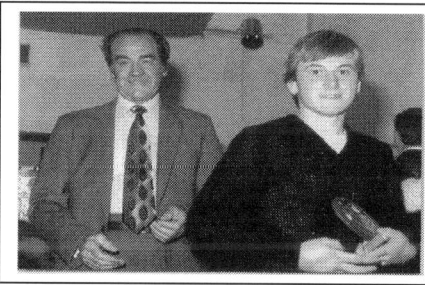 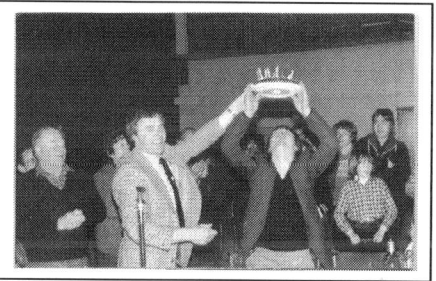

Above

- *On the left - Joe Harvey (Newcastle United legend) presenting me the Player of the Year award at Swan Hunter football presentation evening.*
- *On the right – Geordie Forrest, one of my all-time legends and Swan Hunter football secretary presents me with my 18th birthday cake at Tremblay France. We won the final the following day beating Marseille 1-0. I got the winner direct from a corner (what a flooky goal).*

Swan Hunter Apprentices Football Club Management Team

Chairman	-	Mr Walter Lawrence
Secretary	-	Mr George Forrest
Asst. Secretary	-	Mr Norman Rutherford (also match day sponge man)
Team Manager	-	Tony Mann
Team Coach	-	Derek Hastings *(An absolute legend)*
Committee	-	Mr Ronald Bennet, Mr Cliff Mays, Mr William Bell, Mr Ronnie Lowes

A big thank you to you all, we had some great days and memorable weeks abroad in France and a huge amount of success. Some leaders and some followers but they all played their part (and they done it for nowt)

I actually celebrated my 18th birthday in France and on the day, we were returning to England we had a cup final to play first, which I have already mentioned. After the final we celebrated, like you do,
after winning an international tournament, basically we had a few drinks. I got on the bus for the long journey home feeling a little bit tipsy, wrecked and looking forward to a good kip but as it was my 18th birthday we decided to have a drink and the lads kept topping up my glass. To cut a long story short I can remember asking Jimmy McKeown to get Debbie (now the missus) something big in duty free in case I was to bladdered (drunk). I woke up, what I thought was a few hours later but we had crossed the channel and we were just past Watford gap. Feeling a bit rough I asked Jimmy what he had got Debbie (who was 17yrs old and a stunner, still the same today actually but now she is 52yrs old) anyway he informed me he had got her a massive bottle of Oil of Ulay, I said "your fucking joking Jimmy shell knack me if I give her that", Jimmy said "you said get her something big, so I did".

"Winning isn't everything but losing really sucks"

Anyway, when we got back to Newcastle I headed straight for Fenwick's and got her some posh perfume on tick, four easy payments, to this day she still doesn't know.

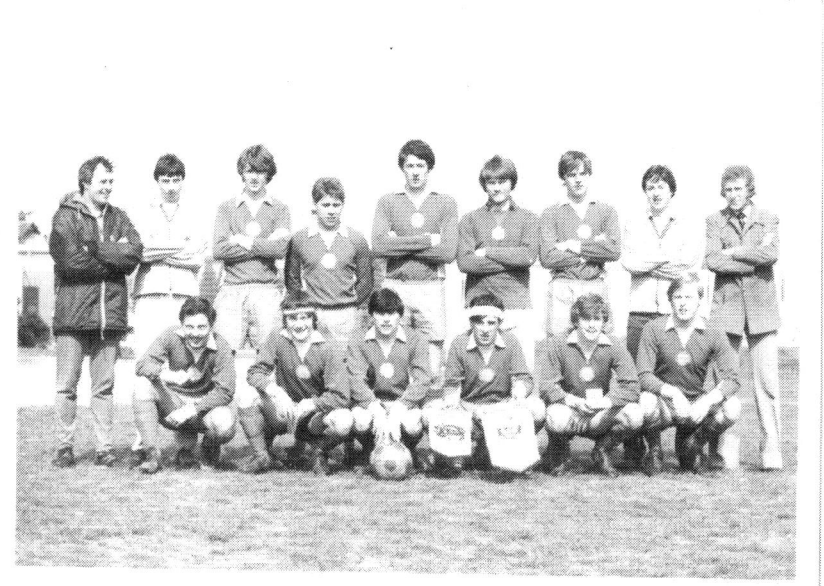

Back row left to right – Geordie Forrest, Brian Hetherington, Jimmy McIntyre, John Cooper, Norman Buglass, Ian McDonald, Paul Baker, Jeff Melstrom, Derek Hastings
Front Row left to right – Paul Harvey, Wally Charlton, Kenny Carr, Ian Bensley, Stevie Senior, Peter McDade

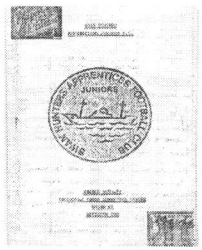

To all the lads at Swan Hunter Football Club

The shipyards maybe no more, but the memories will never die. I have a bad habit of writing poetry (if you can call it that) when I have been inspired, when I am sad/happy or generally when I feel there have been injustice. Here is one of those said poems. Work it out yourself:

Ten years have gone by and what has gone wrong
Wallsend has lost more things than anyone
We used to have Ship yards with ten thousand men
The men have got less, the order books dry
She's going to let the shipyards die
Remember "Haggies" the rope works, it stood through two world wars
But you crushed it "Maggie" with your greedy iron paws
Don't give in people don't let her win
Where Geordies and proud of it, we've been through thick and thin
So fly your blue flag Maggie, let it wave
You'll never send Wallsend to an early grave
June 1986

My time "Doon the yards" was an unbelievable insight into people's behaviours and their role in hierarchy. There was not only hierarchy in the yards but there was also communities and factions you could even call it tribalism and depending on what tribe you belonged to would determine where you sat (literally) in the hierarchy. The tribalism and community aspect is based on what trade or non-trade you belonged to (see below)

"Don't expect success to drop in your hands, work hard, play hard and you may achieve your dreams"

• Caulker burners	• Shipwrights
• Drillers	• Electricians
• Pipe fitters	• Joiners
• Stagers	• Plumbers
• Crane operators	• Platers
• Draughtsman	• Riggers
• Blacksmiths	• Welders
• Paint sprayers	• Labourers
• Store keepers	• Cleaners
• Sheet Metal workers	• Liner offs
• Managers	• Fitters

And apologies for any I have missed.

All trades had bait cabins or sheds scattered across the ship yard. When I say sheds, and cabins I mean mini areas that housed over a hundred blokes and women. If you were a shipwright you ate only in the Shipwrights cabin, a welder in the welder's cabin, you get the point. The only time trades came together was if you ate in the main dinner hall and even then, you sat with your trade. Trades were also separated by different trade unions.

When I first went into the yards as an apprentice I was at the bottom of the pecking order and you were basically a skivvy to your tradesman. You done exactly what he asked you or you got your arse kicked or worse. They were happy to hang you from chain lockers 150ft up in the air, weld your steel toecap boots to the side of the ship, with you in them and place broom shanks or lengths of timber through the arms of your overalls and then hang you from somewhere (imagine the angel of the North) and leave you for a couple of hours, and anything else they felt was appropriate punishment.

I, the good old days, such gentle folk!!!! The bottom line is the yards were a scary place to be but an unbelievable life learning experience. It was like a mini town with shops (blokes selling tabs and sweets from the central stores), bookmakers or blokes who put yu bets on, hospital or dodgy first aid room, restaurants (bait cabins) and a range of communities which were made up of the various trades and finally hard grafting working class people who were the salt of the earth, and just like family's, those blokes who were happy to punish you, were the first to help you out in a crisis, well, as long as it didn't involve work.

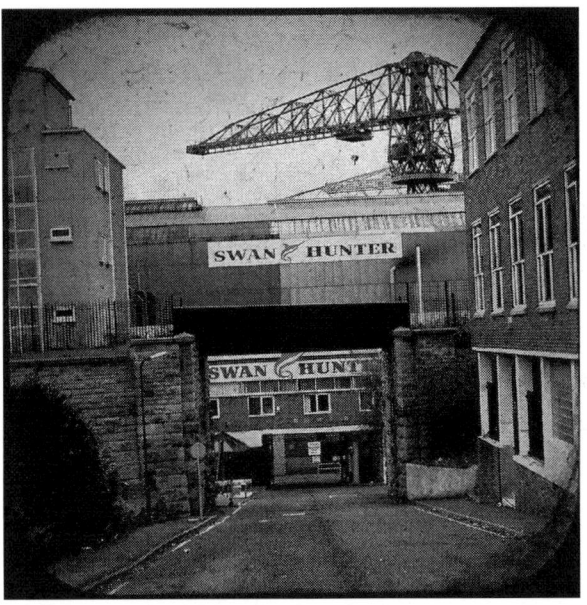

As mentioned earlier, my journeyman was a man called Tommy Moss, hard as nails and built like a brick shit hoos and definitely a bloke you didn't cross. I ended up with Tommy because I was late on the morning when the tradesman chose their apprentices, and everyone avoided Tommy so when I arrived, feeling a bit pissed off because I had been docked a qtr. (15 minutes' pay), Tommy was waiting!!!! The good thing about being Tommy's apprentice was that he had his own cabin with all the mod cons, heaters, stove, kettle, comfy chairs and bunks to get yu heed doon. I have got to say he was also a quality tradesman and knew his job inside out and I learnt a huge amount from a man I grew to respect and admire. He was as fair as they come and looked after me big style. My first two years in the yards were life changing, I learnt how to look after myself, respect and trust the people I worked with, learnt to dodge people in white boiler suits and generally started to become a man. I learnt my trade over the next couple of years and my partner in crime was Roy Murphy, a great lad, he was more laid back than anyone I knew. Our claim to fame was fitting out the officer's galley and levelling the lift decks on HMS Ark Royal and spending two weeks on sea trials, apart from that I can't remember much of the seven years I spent in the yards apart from the knowledge of that working life in the yards was really tough, working in confined spaces or from hundreds of feet in the air, breathing in god knows what shite, being either boiling hot or freezing cold depending on the time of year. I find it amusing when I am sitting in the office I currently work in and people complain that they are too hot, too cold or telling me the servers down and they feel stressed because they can't answer their emails. If only they knew what it was like to work doon the yards.

In summary and to put some context on shipyard working I would say that the modern-day version of team dynamics, culture, hierarchy and delivery of work (organisational development) has changed very little. You had people who are leaders, people who are managers and people who are followers. Internal politics was played within trades and across the organisation and you had to quickly work out who were the plotters and schemers and who were the shirkers and the workers. Bureaucracy was a stumbling block but across trades rather than across organisations. The culture was hierarchical and much more aggressive than today, where unions were strong and very left wing, strikes were common and seemed on some occasions of no value but that was down to my lack of understanding of the national political picture where shipyards were being forced down a route of denationalisation which would result in staff pay offs and more sadly the closure of the shipyards.

The biggest lesson I learnt was don't believe everything you are told until you have the facts to confirm it. In laymen's terms, don't get "shit on" and always protect your back. The other more important lesson was respect, and trust your colleagues and you won't have to worry too much about the sentence above.

I worked in the shipyards in the late seventies and into the eighties and although this was nearly forty years ago I can honestly say that generally the people haven't changed, just the economic, political and technological world we live has changed resulting in people aspiring to new things and I can say that the world today has nearly (but not quite) rid itself of what I call "working class syndrome" where we all knew our place and we were not allowed to get "above our station". Wallsend has created entrepreneurs, pop stars, authors, scientists, doctors, nurses, sporting heroes, war heroes, sea captains, engineers who have helped to develop the third world and god knows how many skilled and academic people, and we even let the Romans build a wal, so don't be too hard on the area, "where deein canny man".

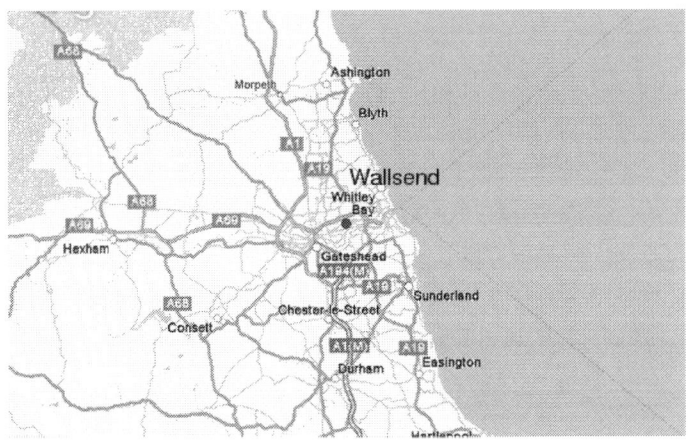

"Be proud of your heritage and never forget where you come from"

Chapter 2

Floggin Kirbys (well who hasn't)

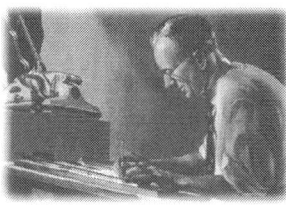 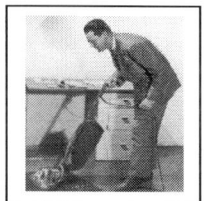

Jim Kirby - Founder

I decided to take my redundancy from the shipyards before they were privatised, and I got a canny little lumpa (redundancy payment) which me and Debbie took little time in spending. I made a decision that I didn't want to return to my trade unless I had to and looked at other opportunities which I always wanted to try. For some strange reason, I always fancied being a salesman. I quite liked the idea of chatting to people and making money from it and working in an office.   I decided to apply for some sales jobs and started with the executive positions, as you do, company car and pension with all the trappings (ive never been a one for setting my sights to low) and very quickly realised that you needed qualifications and experience, so I ended up trying my hand at flogging Kirbys. People of a similar age to me will know the American company I am talking about, but they were based in Newcastle and you needed no experience just enthusiasm. So, I applied and like all the other people who applied, I got the job. No company car or pension and no salary, just commission only, so much for the sales executive but at least I got to wear a suit and tie, which on reflection is just a posh boiler suit.

The interesting thing about this role was I thoroughly enjoyed it and once I had completed the one week's training which consisted of some guy showing us how to use the Kirby and how to do a demo on some carpet and then a breakdown of what we had to say when we were closing a sale with customers. Basically, the higher the price the more we got paid was the outcome of the week and if we didn't flog any then we didn't get any wedge, happy days!!!!!! No union to protect me now and the singing every morning was a bloody nightmare, seriously you had to sing a uplifting rendition of "I'm flogging Kirby's today" or something with all the other salesman, what a hoot.

Anyway, I had arranged some appointments with people who were actually interested in buying these bloody things, so off I toddled in my Vauxhall cavalier (purchased from my redundancy) to meet my very first customer which was a house somewhere in Gateshead. I was shitting my self but quite excited at the same time, I knocked on the door and in I went and started my sales pitch I had been taught (me patta was awaful) but to cut a long story short I flogged the Kirby and made a weeks wages in one sale. I lasted four weeks and in that time I flogged a couple of Kirbys to my family and friends and three to Frankland prison in Durham. I had a mate who worked there and he got me in to do my pitch to his boss and once I had finished he looked at me with a very bland expression and said "give is three" and walked away. I was ecstatic, it was worth a months wages. I decided at the end of the week that I wasn't cut out to constantly put people under pressure, especially working class folk who were watching every penny. Forty eight easy payments or something like that was not my idea of fairness or enjoyment so I walked into the office and told them I was finished. The director of the company invited me into his office and he said "why are you quitting, you have a knack for talking to people, you will make a fortune". I told him that I thought his company was a hell of a place to work but did not fit my pricipals. On reflection I realised that I got my sales because people trusted me quickly and that was down to the fact that I was honest and fair but I was also very good at engaging with people. The company actually celebrated its 100th birthday in 2014 which is one hell of an achievement so well done to all those people who have had that unique experience of floggin a Kirby. You could not have got two contrasting jobs, hairy arsed shipyard worker to bright blue suited salesman but there was a massive learning curve for me in undertaking this role and it was based on values and principals and meeting, talking, negotiating and persuading people to follow my lead and a lot of the people I seen done this. I learnt that people will decide whether they like you within fourteen seconds of meeting you **and that, how you dress, at that time did make a difference.** If I had turned up to those customers in my boiler suit I am certain I wouldn't have got a sale, purely based on peoples impression. The job also taught me that staying true to my principals and beliefs and showing respect and dignity will always overcome lies and deceit. A short chapter in my working life but an important stepping stone to understsnding people, organisations and culture.

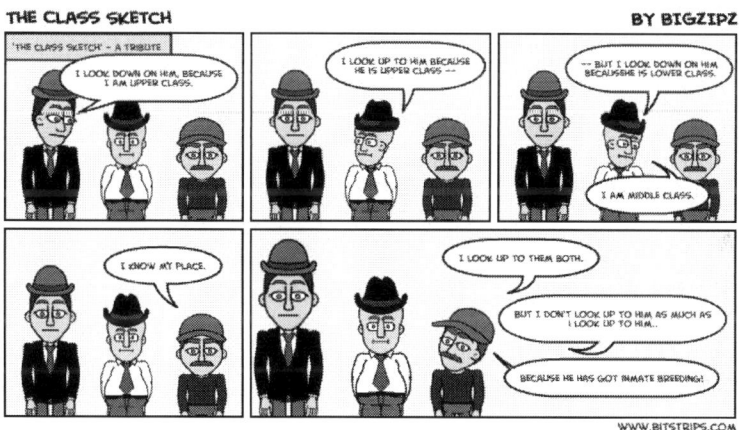

"Working culture varies across the spectrum and you either embrace it or move on, but always reflect on the learning as I guarantee you will come across it again"

Chapter 3

On the Nat King Cole (The Dole)

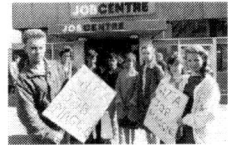 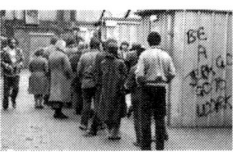 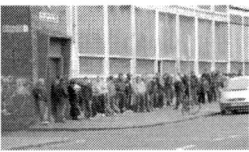

I spent seven months on the dole after leaving Kirby and I can honestly say that I hated every minute of it and I know that the vast majority of people who do have to sign on feel the same. It was the first and only time I was out of work and I vowed that I would never be forced to do it again. I would rather work for myself doing anything at all than have to be treated like the way we were when signing on. Standing in the que with your dole card also known as a UB40, waiting to sign the dotted line to make sure you got your giro made you feel like shite. The punters behind the panel asked the same questions each week, have you undertook any work in the last two weeks, have you applied for any jobs in the last two weeks, are you fit to work and so on. Once the envigorating thirty second interview was over you signed the dotted line and off you toddled with your tail between your legs and a feeling of unusefulness.

The eighties was not a good time to be out of work if you lived in the North East of England. Thatchers Britain was anything within the M25 and if you lived outside of that then you were in bother. She decimated the public sector, shipbuilding industry, privatised anything which had British in front of it and absolutely destroyed the mining industry and communities in the North East. They called her the "Iron Lady". I would not disagree with the statement because she was, in her words "not for turning" but Thatcher and her millionaire ministers had no idea of the pain, suffering, poverty and destruction they caused to this area, actually they did understand what they were doing they just didn't give a shit. Thirty years on and I am still bitter and angry at their deconstruction of the social fabric of this country. My political views are a lot more balanced now as I have got more wiser and experienced life with different governments in power but I will never forgive that horrible, aggressive, conceited and selfish horay henry party. Phew, ive finally got that of me chest.

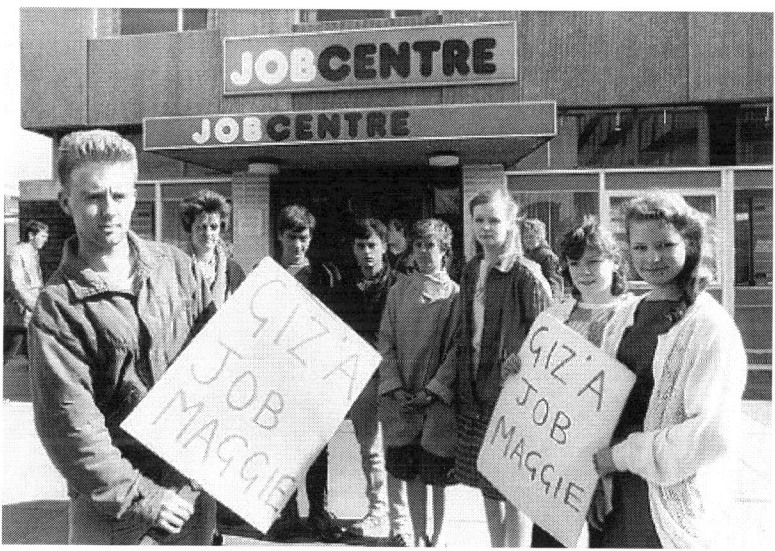

"Margaret Thatcher was not a malicious person. She was a person who couldn't see, or didn't want to see, the unfairness and disadvantaging consequences of the application of what she thought to be a renewing ideology". **Neil Kinnock – Leader of the Labour Party**

Chapter 4

Cleaning Windows with wor kid

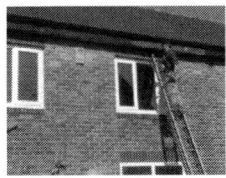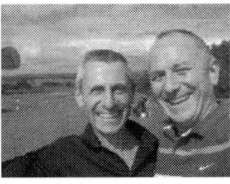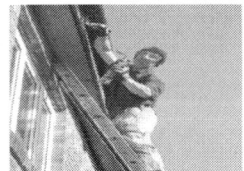

After seven frustrating, soul searching, job seeking, depressing months where I was constantly on the bones of my arse being supported financially by my wonderful wife I decided after a discussion with wor kid that I would clean windows with him. Wor Malc had decided a few years earlier that actually, cleaning windows for a living was a canny little crack, especially after Maggies squad had decided to pay them fifty quid a week for the privilege. I am unbelievably proud of wor Mal for a lot of things but mainly because after thirty years he is still cleaning those same windows today and the customers he has provided a service for are now great friends of his. He has seen generations of family's grow over three decades and he has been a psychologist, counsellor, fixer of drains and roofs, painter of garage doors and windows, snow clearer, prescription collector, taxi driver, supporter of social functions, gardener and furniture maker, gatekeeper and stopper of dodgy salesman and a whole lot more to the vast majority of those customers and their families and not once has he overcharged those people for that service, in fact the vast majority has been free. He is no academic and he will never get a position in the diplomatic corps, but he has served two communities in Wallsend and Cramlington and he is one of the best engagers when talking to people I have seen.

Anyway, that shite above is worth at least a couple of pints or a nice bottle of red off wor kid. There's the context and now here comes my experience. Rather than sit on me arse and feel useless I picked up the bucket with wor kid and started cleaning windows for a living. I thought it would be a doddle, working in the open air, sun on me back, start and finish when I wanted, but how wrong I was. We started eight o'clock sharp every morning, finished at four thirty and then collected until seven pm on a Thursday and Friday and I was deluded with the "sun on me back" comment as most of the time it was bloody freezing. Wor Mal cleaned the top and I cleaned the bottoms. There's a song from Van Morrison called "cleaning windows" and it takes me straight back to this time when I hear it. One of the other things I didn't take into account was that I had to climb over bloody garages to get to the back windows, believe me this was no fun, especially on a cold icy winter's day.

On one such day when it was minus three and brass-monkey cold we both leaned the ladders on the front of the garage, climbed up the ladders and then pulled the ladders on to the garage roof. The roof itself had a layer of ice on it and I would have been more suited skating in Whitley bay ice rink, instead I had the ladders over my shoulder walking slowly across to the back of the garage. Wor kid led the way "watch oot for the ice Wally", "a can bloody see itttttt, shit". Ladders went one way and I went arse over tit, banged me heed and had a huge bruised ego. Wor kid stood there trying desperately to show some concern but instead just burst oot laughing. Anyway, I got up and got to the back of the garage roof, placed me ladders in the back garden and proceeded to climb down, wor Mal was already down and getting ready to clean the top windows. As I started to climb down the ladder it started to slide from the wall, descending slowly onto the garage window making an ear screeching sound as it scraped down the window at which point I slipped on one of the rungs, and landed upside down on the ladder with a twisted knee. I waited for the ladder to go through the window but it didnt. Wor Mals face was a picture of shock and then he tentatively took my weight and helped me of the ladder. "A divvunt think yu cut oot for cleaning windows Wally" and I couldn't agree with him more. It was like a sketch from a Laurel and Hardy movie. I managed to continue on the windows for a good few months after that incident, but I always wanted to work in DIY or sport and when the opportunity came I told wor kid to shuv his bucket and ladder where the sun don't shine and buggard off to pastures new.

In all seriousness, this was one of my best jobs ever, seriously. I was working with not just my brother, but my best mate and we were in control of our destiny. I learnt, apart from how to clean windows with a squeegee, diplomacy, patience and tact when dealing with people and I absolutely appreciated any job thereafter as nothing has been as physically draining as that work. My brother is now fifty-six years old but fitter than most thirty-year olds and he continues to provide a valuable service to those communities. He has made a good living out of his business and his quality of life and work life balance has been exactly how he wants it to be.
The point I am trying to make here is don't underestimate this work and don't devalue similar types of professions, be it shop assistants, factory workers, security workers, cleaners and all other ancillary or retail roles. They are the backbone of this country. Give them a thought on a cold winter's day when the wind is blowing, and you are sitting on your backside getting stressed over the amount of irrelevant emails you have to answer.

"Industry will implode if support workers stop. Windows won't be cleaned, shelves will be empty, and goods won't be delivered, never forget the importance of that work"

Chapter 5

The DIY Shop (Dickens Home improvement hypermarket)

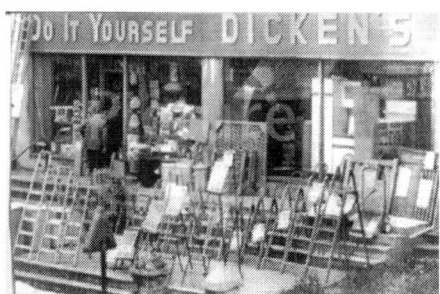

https://picturestocktonarchive.wordpress.com/2005/11/25/dickens-do-it-yourself-store/

After my exploits with wor kid I was lucky enough to get a job in the timber section at Dickens. Although it was only part time it give me and Debbie a little bit income to help pay the bills and keep the wolfs from the door. I was surprised at the size of the shop even though I had visited it on a number of occasions as a customer I obviously never got the opportunity to see what goes on behind the scenes until I started working there. I will never underestimate the level of skill and knowledge retail staff know on products they sell, in fact I thought the job would be a doddle but the amount of knowledge you need to have on the products you have to sell is mind boggling and the staff seemed to know every nut, bolt, type of timber and tool the customer required.

The staff ran the shop like a well-oiled machine with everything in sync and everything in the right place. I learnt about stock ordering using Kanban's (Kanban is a system to control the logistical chain from a production point of view, and is an inventory control system, in simple terms an ordering card for more stock when required), the importance of visual signage and customer engagement and sales. The difference in the store to the shipyards was when you were doing any type of work you done it in front of the customer most of the time which really put you under pressure, especially when you were cutting timber to correct sizes and angles, down the yards you just done it and if you dropped a bollick, you got another piece of timber and done it again. The difference in the store was time and stock was money and in the words of wor Mal "measure twice and cut once" was the way forward. The guys at the store were unbelievably focused and passionate about their roles which surprised me and I was also surprised at the amount of tradesman employed. My impression before I started at Dickens was that the staff were just sales people but that was not the case. I left Dickens after a couple of months to start my next full time job but my time there give me an insight into the dedication and hard work of retail staff. I feel privileged and very fortunate that in my present role I only work Monday to Friday with fantastic holiday entitlement and I don't have to work weekends or bank holidays, can you imagine the state of the economy if all retail outlets done the same? Dickens closed not long after I left (nothing to do with me by the way) but a lot of the staff moved across to what is now B&Q which is currently situated on Middle Engine Lane in Wallsend. One story which sticks in my head was that I worked 4pm til eight most nights and I used to drop of Craig (my oldest son) at my mother and father in-laws. I would usually have a chat and a cuppa and then head off to work but this one time I arrived a little bit late. Jimmy (my father in-law) had made me a cuppa but I said I need to shoot off or I would be late. He said "drink your tea before you go, I chucked some more milk in". I wolfed the tea down and then took the short five-minute drive to work. When I arrived, I got out of the car feeling really sick and then proceeded to spew like hell, I was ill for the rest of the shift and til this day I have never drank tea. A weird and boring story but at least anyone who is reading this will know if they meet me to offer me coffee.

A bit of local history re the emergence of super stores

Over 125 years of history
In 1878, Mr Harry T. Rodgers opened a small ironmongery business in Stockton and in 1925 Alice Dicken, Great Grandmother to Marcus Dicken, the current Managing Director, took over the business. She opened a second shop, managed by her son Harry. In 1960 Albert Dicken, the father of Marcus, entered the company, joining his brothers Robert and Terrence. They moved onto a 1-acre site in Portrack Lane, Stockton, which is now the site of the present At Home Furnishings store. They also purchased a 9-acre farm opposite and began to develop buildings which eventually formed the popular DIY Hypermarket, which attracted thousands of customers from all around the area, as this was the forerunner of today's large DIY stores.

In 1970, Dickens began aggressive TV advertising and, in 1976, ran the first 2-minute TV commercial (with a guest appearance from Marcus Dicken at 6 years old), still a rare event today.
In 1978, the company was bought by the Montague L. Meyer Group and Albert Dicken remained as Chairman. 1980 saw the Shiremoor store opened by Noel Edmonds. Being the TV idol hosting Swap Shop, he attracted thousands of people, causing major traffic jams on all the approach roads. In 1982 Montague L. Meyer merged with International Timber and Albert Dicken purchased the company back in October 1983. The following year, the Washington, Tyne & Wear store was opened, the largest DIY superstore in Europe.

In 1988, Marcus Dicken joined the company and in 1991, Ann joined. Four years later they were married. 1993 saw another link with Noel Edmonds, but this time it was his sidekick Mr Blobby from Noel's House Party. Famous for their Mad, Mad, Mad, Mad January Sales, Dickens booked the mad Mr Blobby to open the sale. Mr Blobby incredibly had the Christmas number one, and again thousands flocked to see this unlikely pop idol.

"If you forget your heritage, you have lost your meaning to progress"

Chapter 6

On the Milk

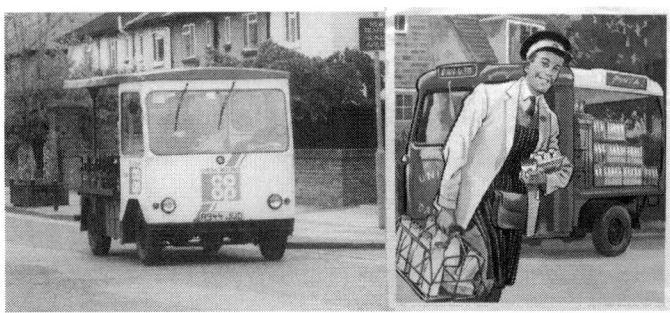

As like a lot of lads my age (fifty plus now) when we were young'uns we got a job as either a milk lad or paper lad to earn some extra wedge. I decided I could do both, so before I trudged of to school I would get up at four in the morning and delivered milk and I was on the milk van for both Bobby Patterson who delivered milk in Howdon and Willington Quay and then Gavin Tyrie who delivered milk in Howdon. It was hard work and you had to be fit and a bit brave as you would hang onto the back of the van whilst Bob or Gavin were giving out their orders of "steri at number four, two pints at number six" and so on. The van very rarely stopped so you were basically shuttling back and forth from the van and the houses trying desperately to keep up with the bloody jabbering orders of Bob or Gavin. We worked from 5am to about 7.30am then dived in the hoose, quick wash, school uniform on and off to school, Willington High in my case. It was bloody hard to graft yu bollicks off for three hours on the milk and then go to school and try and learn something without falling asleep, which I did on many occasions, but at least I left school with some qualifications.

Anyway, I had already experienced early mornings when I was young so when I was offered a full-time job at Co-Operative creameries at west street, Wallsend I was over the moon. I was asked to take on the milk round in walker which was great fun and I loved the round. Once you had loaded up your crates of milk, pop, eggs and yoghurts you were out of the depot and onto the empty roads of Wallsend and Walker. Believe me when I say the work was tough, mentally and physically, just trying to remember me route was difficult, never mind trying to remember what bottles of milk went where but after a month or so I knew every single door on my round and who got what on what day. It was fantastic in the summer but absolutely shite in the winter apart from Christmas when you got your tips and believe me I needed them as me and Debbie were on the bones of our arses. The bairns wanted for nowt (never spoilt them though) but me and Debbie had to graft as much as we could to just keep our heads above water, so much so that I also had a part time barman's job on an evening at Wallsend Supa snooker (The Miners club), honestly, we were knackered every day, like a lot of other people who were in the same boat. My customers were great, and I got to know them well, the experience of working with wor Mal on the windows and the work I had done previously give me loads of confidence when dealing with some customers who still wanted their deliveries but weren't that keen on paying. I have got to say the Walker people are the salt of the earth, densely populated working-class area with all the inner city social issues to go with it but very proud and hardworking people who don't beat about the bush, they just tell you how it is. The one thing I can say about working in the early hours on a council estate is you see and experience some things which you wouldn't probably see later in the day. I regularly give lifts to drunken customers who were heading back from the toon after a night oot and on more than one occasion captured people having it away at the bottom of their stairs, a quickie before he headed off to work, or in the arches of some of the houses, my reaction was usually "morning, yu alreet" and then I cracked on. Getting yu milk deliveries nicked was also common and sometimes it was other milkmen who were doing it which caused some

35

barneys between the milk man fraternity. Any opportunity to get extra customers and by any means was a regular occurrence. Mmm "Milk wars", canny name for another book.

Delivering milk can be a lonely experience and if the shit hits the fan you have to sort it, you're on yu tod, nee mobile phones if yu were in bother, in fact yu were lucky to find a phone box with the phone still working. This role taught me, as stupid as it may sound to make quick and effective decisions and it also taught me the importance of lone working and the dangers that come with that. People paid for their milk in either cash or tokens and you collected that money on a daily basis and Thursday and Friday evenings, I wouldn't have been the first bloke who had the shit kicked out of him for his leather money bag wrapped around his shoulder but fortunately, although I had a few close calls it never happened to me.

For some strange reason, some of my family, namely my wife Debbie, sister Bev, brother Mal and sister in-law Andrea all wanted to experience delivering milk, so I arranged for them to come out with me, not al togetha like yu naa, at different times. So, I will explain very quickly their little trip out on the electronic milk float and the things they said and done. My wife and sister, who to this day are as thick as thieves, said they both wanted to come out with me as they thought it would be fun!!! Once we got out on the round I started to tell them to put a pint here and a steri there and after about thirty minutes they said they would just sit in the cab as it was a bit cold. I always used to stop halfway on my round, usually by the Byker wall and have a quick cup of coffee and a fag, no more than ten minutes. Anyway, we stopped, and our Bev pulled out this huge picnic basket which was full of sarnies, pork pies, crisps, cheese, chocolate bars and the biggest flask I had ever seen. I looked in amazement and said, "what the hell have yu got there, wu only stopping for five minutes", she said "well I thought we could have a little picnic", "am delivering bloody milk man not taking a stroll in the country". She then turned to me and Debbie, and with a big sigh said, "a can't believe it, I've forgot the milk for wu cup of coffees", seriously, she did. Me and Debbie looked at each other then I told her to turn around as there was seventy gallons behind her, what a hoot.

Next to come out was wor Mal. He, like me worked on the milk when he was younger, and he said he fancied coming out to see if it was still the same crack. It was a Saturday morning when he decided to come out and he was late, he was supposed to be meeting me at wor house and then we would head of to the dairy, but he didn't turn up and I was now running late so I just went without him. I got to the dairy and loaded the float as quick as I could then I was off. I pulled out the depot and there was wor kid sitting on the wall with the clothes he had on from the night before and it became apparent why, he still hadn't been yem and he was pissed as a fart after a night oot at the coast. I told him to jump in the cab and say nowt until I got on the estate. He just looked at me with a drunken smile and said "wey I, nee bother Wal" and then put his heed back and went to kip. He woke up three hours later just as I was finishing me round with a dazed and confused look, "mek es a cuppa man wor kid, me mooth tastes like a camel rider's sock". I just shook me heed made him a cuppa and headed back to the dairy and wor kid jumped in the car whilst I unloaded the empties and we then headed home.

The final wannabee was wor Andrea. She was bloody hyper and unbelievably excited, and I've got to say she grafted like hell for a couple of streets and then decided to sit the rest of the round out. She did ask if she could have a quick drive of the float and I thought well she can't do much harm it's just like driving a dodgem car, one pedal to accelerate and one pedal to stop. I told her to just press the pedal gently to accelerate and to do the same with the other pedal when she was stopping. She took nee notice at all and slammed her foot doon. The float shot forward as I was thrown back shouting "stop, stop" so she proceeded to slam her foot on the brake and the float came to an immediate stop. I can remember the silence; there was no one around as it was only five thirty in the morning and the only sound was the rattle of milk bottles and the tweeting of the birds as the crates swayed forward and back. I sat, waiting for the crash of the crates and bottles but they rocked back and forward and then came to a stop. Andrea just burst out laughing "that was great", I looked at her with a shocked face and told her to sit in the passenger seat and don't touch anything. None of the above people ever came out with me again but we all have a good laugh remembering those events.

After delivering milk for six months I was offered the post of stock controller (posh title eh) for the depot, which basically meant loading all the milk vans at the dairy and checking that the blokes weren't fiddling. I also replenished the cold store and offloaded thousands of gallons of milk from an articulated lorry every day, I was as fit as a butcher's dog and I was a little bit warmer being in the depot.

The next time you buy a bottle/carton of milk just give a little thought to the people who are delivering it to either the shops or your front door. Think about the unsociable hours they work, the weather they have to deal with and the stressful deadlines they are working to, yes deadlines, if you haven't got milk for your cornflakes in the morning you know you will be pissed off when you head of to work. The old dairy on West Street and the blokes who worked there have now gone but that place sits deep in the heritage of this area and provided milk to the masses in Wallsend and Walker. I play golf at Wallsend golf club and when I tee off from the par three thirteenth which runs alongside west street I always have a little look up at the residential home which now fills the Wallsend dairy land and have myself a little smile as I remember fondly those cold mornings delivering milk.

"Certain memories, sounds, smells, remind you of times in your life, treasure them or dismiss them"

Chapter 7

Voluntary work

Willington Quay and Howdon Boys Club

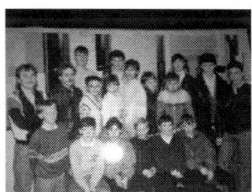

I worked as a volunteer at Willington Quay and Howdon Boys Club and more recently Newcastle East End Football Club. My time at Willington Quay and Howdon was at the very start of my working life and I went on to become the club leader which I was paid a small amount of money per month. The work at the club was very close to my heart as my father, uncles and brothers were all members of the club in the 50s and 60s representing the club at football. The club was part of my community and it was a place of enjoyment and fun for loads of kids who are now adults and have children of their own. I have many memories of the club and the people who worked there with me and the members who attended.

Steve Johnson, Jeff Millen and Gary McEwen were three dedicated and passionate workers who provided a huge amount of their time to the club. I regularly speak to the lads and lasses and chat about some of the great times we had. Our adventure weekends to Billsmoor in Otterburn, Northumberland, the football team, the trip to Alton towers and the many, many events and competitions we attended at the club and all over the country. If there was a free trip being offered from Northumberland association of Boys Clubs, we were the first ones to offer our services. The most memorable moments I had of my time at the club was the Christmas shows we put on for the community. I can honestly say all those lads and lasses from the age of eight to twenty years old were an absolute credit to their families and the community. Yes, we had all the social problems, drugs, alcohol, poverty, unemployment but these guys never let anyone down, especially their community. Take a bow, every single one of you. My voluntary work at the club give me the opportunity to start to understand the meaning of community work and what it really meant, it also allowed me to commence my career as a community development worker.

During this period of my working life a disaster took place *which was horrific and avoidable, and I had to right about it. I wrote the poem below a couple of days after the tragedy. The Herald of Free Enterprise* was a roll-on roll-off ferry which capsized moments after leaving the Belgian port of Zeebrugge on the night of 6 March 1987, killing 193 passengers and crew. The poem is called:

"Money before safety"
They all left the port in merry cheer
Sipping their wine and drinking their beer
No one could imagine the horror ahead
So many people were going to be dead
The ship turned one way then the other
Back again and it was over
Children were screaming people were crying
The disaster had started, people were dying
So many lives lost as it hit the sea bed
This is what the hierarchy had always dread
What about the ship owners, they knew the score?
So many lives lost through a fault in the door
They're not interested in the people who were lost
They're only interested in the ship and the cost
Wally Charlton – March 1987

"Don't be a do gooder, be a good doer"

Newcastle East End Football Club

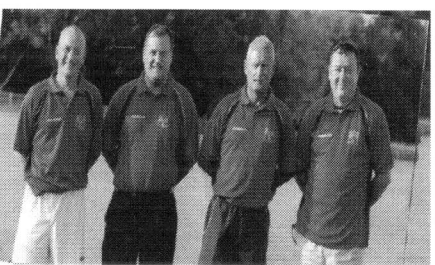

From left to right – Me, Kelly Scott, Charlie Scott and Dave Latimer

My more recent voluntary work has been with Newcastle East End Football. I first started there when Gary (my nephew) started playing for the u12s which was the first team in NEEFCs history which commenced in 1995.

Gary was the first of a number of Charlton's to play for the club, Craig and Liam (my sons), Andrew (wor Mals son) and Laura (wor bevs daughter and Gary's sister) have all played for the club. Gary also went on to coach a very successful team which Liam and Andrew were part of. I started to pull some funding applications together for the club with some success and before I could say "howay the lads" I was coaching one of the teams. I still do a little bit of work for the club; I've really got no choice as my sister is now married to my wonderful brother in law Charlie Scott who is the co-founder of the club, along with his son Kelly who I am great friends with. The team I ran were a great set of lads who we took to America on tour, what an experience that was. The lads were all staying with families from the club who hosted our stay, Quincy FC, which is in the state of Illinois. We arrived in Quincy in 100-degree heat which was a shock to the system for these lads from Walker

"Your actions are your responsibility, use them wisely"

and Wallsend. We spent ten days playing games around the state and we also developed a scholarship programme with Quincy University where some lads from the club studied over the next few years. It was a trip of a lifetime for me and the lads and when I bump into the likes of Steve Mason, big Mark and Fraser and all the other lads we immediately reminisce to the trip. I ended up becoming the funding officer at the club which created a number of opportunities for the members of the club.

Dave Latimer who has been at the club for fifteen years sums the history of the club up a lot better than me (see below)

Back in the 1890s two rival Northern League amateur sides were top dogs up in the North East. One of those teams was Newcastle East End FC, a team formed in 1881 by a local cricket club (Stanley FC) and the name East End was created in 1882 to avoid confusion with the Durham town of Stanley.

East End FC were one of the founder members of the Northern League. Newcastle East End FC was the first club from Newcastle to go professional in 1889 which was a huge step in those days!

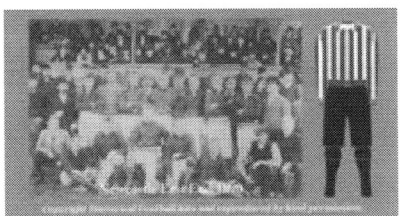

A great read to see the pitch locations of Stanley / East End FC can be found in an article by Paul Brown – "Before St James' Park: the origins of Newcastle United" published in February 2011.

Their closest rivals across the city were Newcastle West End and it was their financial difficulties which set the ball rolling for talks and eventual merger between the two clubs in 1892 to what is now known as Newcastle United FC.

Now NUFC as we all know play in black and white, however it was East Ends red and white kit they used for the first two years of existence, something they would never consider now I am sure! In fact the rivalry with Sunderland is so strong when Puma agreed to sponsor NUFC in 2010 their trademark black Panther was changed to white!)

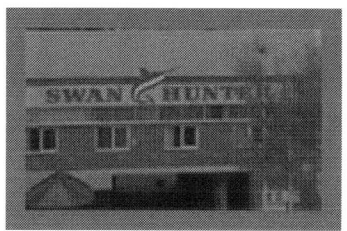

Roll forward almost 100 years later to 1995, and a father and son decide to re-launch the famous Newcastle East End and build the club up from the grassroots.

Charlie and Kelly Scott set about, with the support of Newcastle City Council, to form Newcastle East End Juniors & Seniors FC – the phoenix had risen from the ashes!

The club started with only one junior team however over the last 15years they have established themselves as one of the most respected local clubs in the region and have progressed up the Football Association accreditation scheme to become one of only a handful of **FA Charter Standard Community Club** status in Newcastle.

The club boasts teams with a mix of Minisoccer, junior boy and girls teams, Under 19s and both Male and Female adult teams and a disability team. The next phase of development is well underway as they look to develop a disabled section within the club.

Their venue is one to be admired as they have 5 pitches, all with drainage, changing rooms, clubhouse and lounge to accommodate over 400 members and their parents, family and spectators. The club have reverted back to the original name of the venue also, **Swans Recreation Ground**, which as the name suggests was the venue for the workers at Swans to relax and play sports.

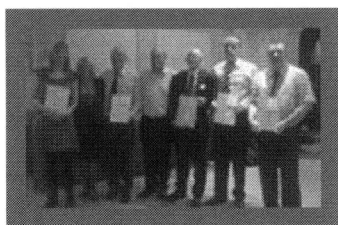

If you want to find out more about East End you may: Email: info@newcastleeastend.co.uk

Newcastle east end football club have fifty plus volunteers who spend on average of ten hours a week coaching, doing admin, working in the kitchen, organising transport and if you do the sums (based on the national minimum wage) they provide £162k per year of free service. This calculation has no on costs etc so add another 20% to the total and you have approximately £200k per year. Not a bad saving for the government. This is the minimum amount, and I know that the likes of Charlie, Kelly and a lot of the other volunteers are at that club seven days a week. The vast majority of these volunteers are in full time employment with jobs ranging from chief executive, self-employed, nurses, academics and retail staff and tradesman. These people do it because they see the difference they are making to the kids and the adults at the club and the benefits it has for the community of Walker and Wallsend.

"When you are questioning why you do it; just reflect on what you have achieved"

Now I'm going to get a little bit political and unfortunately, have a pop at the FA and other local and national funding bodies. Why do these people and other similar organisations make voluntary organisations jump through bureaucratic funding hoops to be awarded poultry sums of money to keep the club afloat? For god's sake Newcastle East End has over five hundred members who don't just play football they do a whole range of social activities. Why can't the funders award these organisations on what they are providing? Why can't the group of people awarding the funding go to the club and see how they operate and look at what they provide instead of sitting in a room and making a decision on what could quite easily be a load of bullshit. I write funding bids and I have been very successful both as a professional and a volunteer. Write what they want to hear and make sure you meet the criteria and you are in with a good chance of success. I understand the process of accountability and governance re any funding regime and why we need to target certain areas and people, but the majority of these organisations are trying desperately to do this, that's why they do what they do!!!!

They're bloody volunteering in their community because they want to make a difference, there passionate about helping people who, for whatever reason need some support but they didn't realise that they had to play politics and have a clear understanding and knowledge of writing funding applications. I know there are people employed in the local authority, The FA and other national and local funding bodies to monitor and administer applications but instead of employing these people to check that the correct box has been ticked and the criteria has matched. Get out to the groups and make a decision based on the reality of what they are seeing and what is needed rather than what the funders feel they should have.

I find it sickening when I see the FA pontificating on sky sports or one of the radio stations about what they have done for grassroots football when actually, they have achieved, in my opinion, very little at all in comparison with the likes of Spain, Holland, Sweden etc.

They provide a number of courses where you either have to travel to or they cost a substantial amount of money so if you are good at writing bids you will have the money to do this but if you are struggling, there is a good chance you're getting nowt and you're either paying for it yourself or you have to fundraise through bag packs, raffles and domino cards etc. which, in most cases is money towards materials, kit and the running of the club.

I am aware that everything costs but should it always be the volunteer who must pay. Give these people a break, they are providing a wonderful service the vast majority of the time and they are doing it for free and they have got their police checks, accounts and constitution in order. Give them a tenth of the £200k they provide free and they will be delighted. Look on any FA website for available courses and they will provide you with a bloody load of them and I have no doubt they are delivered by well qualified and experienced people. The next thing you will see, usually in bold is where cheques have to be paid to but try and find the cost, it's a bloody nightmare.

If the FA, who I have no doubt are passionate about the sport, want grassroots football to develop and provide all the national strategic targets they talk about then change the way you operate.

Just to be clear, all the organisations above provide a fantastic service for voluntary organisations, but they sometimes get lost in their own laborious bureaucracy which slows things down and frustrates the bloody life out of the people delivering the front line service.

The culture of most voluntary organisations is very similar to that of mainstream organisations. They have rules and regulations to follow, guidelines and governance and financial responsibilities which creates systems and processes similar to any public or private sector culture, but the slight difference is the "can do attitude" and the passion and drive to make a success of what they have, knowing that if they fail they will close down.

"Football is a simple game, stop complicating it!!!!!"

There is also more freedom to make rational decisions without having to present to a number of committees, managers and hierarchy. Us so called professionals could learn a lot from how these organisations operate. How do they deal with conflict; how do they stay afloat without being bailed out and how do they manage budgets? Some time spent in the "real world" may help us change how we operate and provide services re access and funding, after all said and done they are providing a service to the same people health or social care provide.

Football Scouting

Through my voluntary work at the club I was offered the opportunity to become a football scout for Newcastle United FC. Peter Kirkley was the development officer at NUFC at the time and he offered me the position. He has been involved in junior football for as long as I can remember and as a young'un I played for him for Wallsend BC. Anyway, I worked at NUFC for a couple of seasons and enjoyed every minute. I was out three or four evenings a week and most weekends looking at potential talent across North Tyneside, Newcastle and Northumberland. It's fair to say that there are plenty of talented players out there, but it is less apparent than it was ten years ago. I would also say that I am not a firm believer in taking kids as young as seven years old to a professional football club where they have to give a huge amount of commitment attending a number of training sessions and games per week, in my opinion denying them their childhood. The opposite viewpoint is the opportunity presented to them is massive and life changing with the dream of becoming a professional footballer. All professional football clubs are competing for the best players and they are getting younger and younger which I think is affecting the grassroots game. Take kids to clubs at thirteen/fourteen years old and see how they develop.

Note for parents, the commitment on your behalf is huge and please do not make the assumption that your child has "made it" because they are at a professional club, the long, long journey has just begun so either enjoy the ride and deal with the very likely possibility of disappointment for you and your child or deny your child the opportunity, what a bloody difficult decision to make.

After my two seasons at NUFC I decided I wasn't enjoying the brief I had been asked to follow regarding recruitment of players, so I left. I had a short spell at Hartlepool United, but I didn't have the same commitment, so I decided to pack it in. If you ever get the opportunity to undertake a scouting role, take it, it is a remarkable rewarding and eye-opening experience.

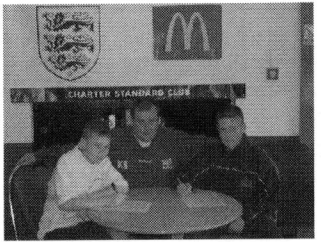

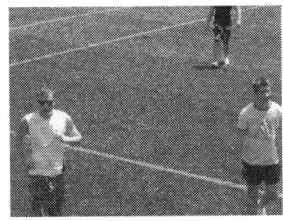 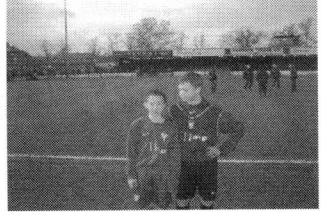

"If you want to be a professional footballer then work hard, train hard, be respectful to others and be prepared for knock backs and disappointment".

Chapter 8

Fundraising with the lads

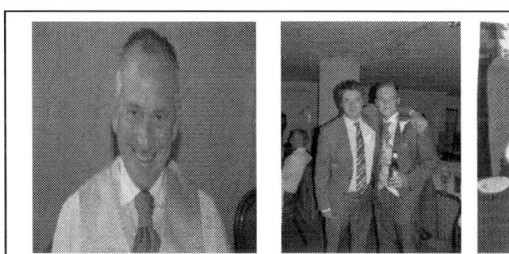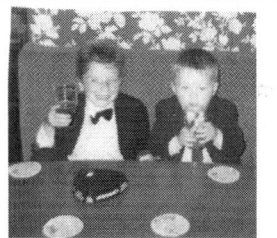

Above - Left to right, Me, the auld bloke, in the middle photo Gary and Craig at Craig's wedding and right, Craig and Gary at their Aunty Andrea and Uncle Jason's wedding, they were having business meetings from a really early age and they've always liked a pint!!!.

Since my very early voluntary days I have been fundraising either to trusts or organising events, raffles etc. and I have had some reasonable successes. Fast forward twenty or so years and I continued to fund raise but now as a volunteer at Newcastle East End FC. We were fortunate to have some real success with our funding, both with small and large pots of money (£2k up to £900k) but we all worked bloody hard to pull the bids together and then deliver a whole range of community and football related projects. This lead to other football clubs contacting me for some advice on achieving funding success.

To cut a long story short, initially Gary and I started a business consultancy called IFC4All and we very quickly developed a data base of over four hundred sporting clubs across the northern region. We both attended an entrepreneur's course at Sunderland University through the Business Innovation Centre and then received some funding to kick start the business. The consultancy was reasonably successful, but I knew we were pissing of some of the FAs and funding bodies because we were undertaking some of the work which they wanted to do but they were not that keen on meeting clubs most week nights between 7-10pm, but we were. Anyway, for a number of reasons we decided to moth ball the business and then Craig kick started the business again a few years later with the support of Gary and me and again we were reasonably successful. We wound the business up due to the lack of time we had to develop the bids. We were doing this on top of our full-time roles and it was becoming impossible to juggle both. We started this consultancy because we were, and we still are passionate about grassroots football. The money we charged barely covered our expenses (we charged 10% - No funding no fee basis), it wasn't irrelevant, but the most important aspect of the work was showing organisations that they can sustain their club and develop it into something very special by developing clear concise and simple funding and development strategies.

The dynamics of running a business with family members are different to just running a business. Sometimes the waters can get muddied and I think we definitely experienced this aspect, but I can honestly say that it was a great experience. Just for the record lads, count me out of anything you want to do re business ventures, I just want to chill oot with the free time I have after a day's graft.

Chapter 9

Working for the Council

It was through my voluntary work that I was offered a position with North Tyneside Council as a play worker. Initially based at Longbenton play centre and then the Meadowell estate. I worked on the estate for five years with some great people and we delivered some great work to the kids from the estate. We worked in different parts of the estate. The outdoor play site, The Barn, The book centre, Collingwood youth club, Luton crescent and The Cedarwood as well as the holiday play schemes. Here is a little bit of poetry from some of my experiences on the estate. The first is based on a residential weekend (which we done once every couple of month)

The Netherton Nightmare
Away I go on an early Friday night
My son and my wife are a distant sight
Two days of torture is what we've got
I miss Craig and Deb a hell of a lot
Fridays nearly over I'm ready for my bed
It feels so strange without Craig and Deb
I wake up Saturday morning to a hell of a site
There's been quite a lot of damage during the night
My morale is low my enthusiasm nil
I hope the warden doesn't call the old bill
We've decided to take two kids home

The rest of them grumble and start to moan
When I get back to my three-bedroomed semi
And they get back to their screw driver and gemi
I think I'll sit down and have one hell of a scream
Then I will realise that play work is not my scene

The above poem is based on a weekend residential with a group of teenage lads and lasses to discuss why they TWOC?? (Taking without owner's consent). Although the weekend was a nightmare I learnt to understand why people do what they do and why, in some cultures there is a total lack of understanding of the harm, hurt and disruption they cause by doing what they do. These group of people thought that what they did was the norm and that they were entirely in their rights to nick cars and motorbikes. I could say that these young people were socially disadvantaged and that they were never given opportunities we might have experienced, probably true, but to be quite honest I would be talking rhetorical bullshit if I was to try and justify their actions. The bottom line is that they knew exactly what they were doing but they didn't really care about the consequences. Call me old fashioned but I just think they had little or no respect for anybody. Don't get me wrong, I am a strong believer in social justice and I firmly believe that we need to give everyone the opportunity to prosper and to take opportunities when they present them to us all, but regardless of your social status we all must stay within the law. The Netherton escapade was a blip in the time I spent on the estate as the vast majority of the people were hard working and caring people who wanted the best for their families.

In my time at the council I had a number of roles, some by choice and some forced upon me through re-structure after re-structure. My roles included play worker, events manager and community development worker with the last one being the most enjoyable and rewarding role. I don't want to get in to the individual roles, so I am going to talk about the organisation and jump into the roles when necessary.

Working in a political and ever-changing environment is unbelievably frustrating and creates no sustainability for worker or the public but unfortunately that is the way political cycles work and the staff are the pawns in a complex game of political chess which does not always result in the best outcome for the people of the borough. My experience in the council was having to play a never ending political justification game. I am aware that times have changed, and this may not be the case now but I am happy to debate with anyone that that was the case then. Sixty local councillors with the majority being labour and then the Tories and the liberals.

What an assortment of people. A mixture of power trippers, bullshitters, know-alls and normal passionate community focused people who wanted to make a positive difference to people's lives. The trouble was they politicised just about everything we did. Sometimes for the right reasons but sometimes because their egos got the better of them. If I opened a kids club up in one ward (with all the relevant justification) I would inevitably be challenged by other councillors re why I hadn't done the same in their ward. The bottom line was that I really couldn't give a shit about their pathetic egotistic political point scoring I just wanted to give children and young people the opportunity to play safely. I must add that this was not the norm, but I can remember one incident where I opened a kid's club in a so called affluent area, there was a need and every child has the right to play regardless of their social status. Anyway, once this kids club opened I was hauled through the coals by my senior manager for opening a service in an area which did not support the political party he was attached to. If I am being honest I knew I would be bollicked by him, but I also knew there was a need and it was a good use of public money. I also made sure there was plenty of press associated with the opening which made it impossible for the said political puppet to close it.

On another occasion, I was asked to leaflet drop for a prospective local candidate. I said, "sorry I can't do that in work time its illegal", I was told "you will do it, I'm your manager" I told him to either suspend me or piss off and get some other puppet to do his dirty work. I wasn't suspended but I was definitely off the Christmas card list. The irony is that I had been leaflet dropping for that candidate but in my own time.

This same guy had asked me to undertake a funding review at a local and very active community group who weren't shy saying exactly what they felt, and they were not saying very nice things about their local councillors. I went to the group and sat with the members, who I had developed good working relationships with over a number of years. The result of my review, which I let the group know first, was a continuation of their funding but with a reduction in some areas which was based on my findings.

The group were happy with this but when I presented my report to this numpty he pushed another report in front of me for the same group, but this report stated that they were not receiving any funding. He then told me to sign it, hahaha "im not signing that, do you think im stupid, you sign it". He went absolutely ballistic, telling me my career was finished, and I wasn't a team player. My response was, and sorry for repeating myself, "sack me or piss off", he stood up and leaned his huge frame over me and told me I was fucked, and actually, I knew I was, so that same week I applied for voluntary redundancy and I got it. Within a week I was gone. There is a tale of how I got my redundancy so quickly, but I will not be able to tell that story until I retire!!

Working for the council was an unbelievable experience with some really high points but some very low points as well, some of my own making I must add. I was fortunate to work with some great people, both colleagues and councillors from all parties. All the guys at the events unit who delivered some great events for the people of North Tyneside and further afield, Fish Quay festival and the International Football tournament to name just two, and my mentor, mate and minder, the most caring and compassionate person you will ever have the pleasure to meet, Gladys Wilson.

My experience of working for the council is that it can be an aggressive, frustrating and a bureaucratic environment to work in, but it also offers employees autonomy and creativity to deliver.

"Change is the only thing that won't change in the public sector"

Over the past ten years the council have been ravaged with cut after cut and a huge amount of their services have now been out sourced to private companies with the staff having to make that move, at least the ones who haven't either taken or been made redundant. The future for the council does look bleak and I can only see more efficiency savings!!!! (Cuts in real terms) continuing.

It is without doubt a political environment but for good reason, that is the main role of the council, to govern the borough through political processes which have been endorsed by voters and if I have any advice for anyone wanting to move into this field I would suggest you are prepared to be of strong character and see change as an opportunity and not a threat.

Time for a poem (tongue in cheek take re tourist info for North Tyneside)

Come to North Tyneside and enjoy yourself
Breathe that sea air; it's good for your health
There's Whitley Bay, Tynemouth and Cullercoats to
All of them have a splendid sea view
Glorious by day, beautiful at night
The castle, the plaza and St Marys light
Plenty to do for young and for old
Sometimes warm and not that cold!!!
So come to North Tyneside, give it a crack
You'll love it so much you'll want to come back
Wally Charlton 1990ish

"Challenge your councillors, they are working for you and you should never let them forget that"

Chapter 10

Kids Party world (Booncey castles and face painted kids)

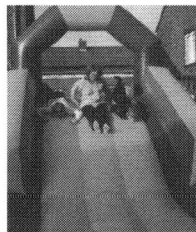

Love this picture of Debbie, Craig and Liam, testing one of the castles

When I left the council, I didn't have a bloody clue what I was going to do, so I travelled down to Hull and purchased four booncey castles and one inflatable slide, using the vast majority of my redundancy money. Although I felt in control of my destiny I was shittin myself because I had no idea if this business venture would work. I had two young lads and a mortgage to pay for and a wonderful wife who not only supported what I was doing but also worked full time to try and ease the financial pressure I had put us in. I take my hat off, and I genuinely respect people who go out on their own. No bugga to sort yu tax, insurance out and if your ill, well tough shit, you have to work. I do get irritated with some people who have the privilege, and it is a privilege having six weeks paid annual leave or more, union support and sickness pay and they still fuckin moan, they have no idea!!!!

The plan for the business was to provide a one stop shop for children's parties, clowns, venue, and castles, face painting, you get the picture, and it worked, for a short period of time. It was really hard work and trying to pull the packages together was enjoyable but not worth my while financially, so I decided to just hire out castles and it was great fun. I hired one or two out during the week and then on a weekend it was all systems go. All the castles would be out, and Craig and Liam would give me a hand to set them up at the venues and that was such a thrill for me. The other benefit for the lads was during the holidays and on weekends when it was a bit slow I would just put one of the castles up in the back garden and Craig, Gary, Liam and their mates would spend the whole day playing on them. I can honestly say they loved the fact that they had these castles on call at any time. The rest of the family (the adults) also had a great time playing on them, usually puggled (drunk), but good fun all the same. After twelve months, I decided I had to get something a bit more financially stable just so we could eat and pay the bills, so I started to apply for some jobs I fancied but I was only after part time work as I was still running the business. Working for yourself can be a very, very lonely place both financially and mentally but what I missed most was the lack of interaction with colleagues. I always work better around other people. It helps me generate ideas and enthusiasm and people generally tell you when you are on the right track or your thinking/idea is just not worth pursuing. Either way people who are sitting whinging about their colleagues or bosses need to take a step back and reflect that they have the opportunity to whinge, poor Debbie was the one who got all mine. The upside was meeting so many wonderful people who regardless of their social or financial status wanted to celebrate their child's birthday or celebration in style.

The plan for the business in my dream world, and this was more than fifteen years ago (ive still got the business plan) was to develop a multi-purpose static venue which had facilities for children's parties which provided catering and also a play area and training venue. Fast forward fifteen years and they are popping up all over the place. If anyone has a spare five hundred grand they want to invest I have a plan which will make millions!!!, seriously I have.

A really funny story (although a bit scary and dangerous at the time) which I have just remembered. Whilst working for the council we were setting up one of our many community events we delivered and on this bright and sunny Saturday summer morning we had four different events running.

"Don't reflect on what you can't change, focus on where you can make a difference"

 It was my job to go to all four sites and make sure the play villages (loads of booncey castles) were set up safely and correctly. I arrived at one of the sites bright and early (7.30ish) just as the event staff were laying out the castles and roping of the village. I was concerned that there was a strong breeze whipping across, not enough to stop the event but enough to make me slightly nervous. Joking aside, these things are lethal weapons and fatalities have occurred because of castles not being tethered down correctly or inflating a castle in strong winds.

I made sure all the staff had tethered the castles down correctly (we hammered, at an angle, metal spikes about three feet long into the ground to hold the castle in place). Once this was done I was happy that things were in place, the staff were also aware that if the wind picked up they would drop the castles. I jumped in the van and made a few phone calls and after about five minutes I heard some shouting from where the castles were and when I looked up there was a 20ft x 20ft castle bouncing freely across the field and heading for our children's entertainers, who for some strange reason decided they could stop it. They stood in a star like position with their feet planted to the ground and actually tried to stop the castle. "Fuck me" was the cry as I jumped out of the van and across the field. The castle just stormed over the entertainers like a steamroller and came to a stop at a garden fence.
Although this was unbelievably dangerous and horrific to watch it was also so comical. I ran straight to the people who had been flattened and they were both in a "snow angel" position on the ground. Although a bit shocked they had no injuries which I was so pleased to see.   When we investigated the

incident, it came too light that one of the events staff had decided to change the pins when the castle was inflated which is a definite NO, NO. They were never asked to work another event and the children's entertainer continues to entertain kids across the North East, happy days.

"Never under estimate the power of mother nature, she will bite your arse at any given time"

Chapter 11

The Millennium Man (working for Blyth Valley council)

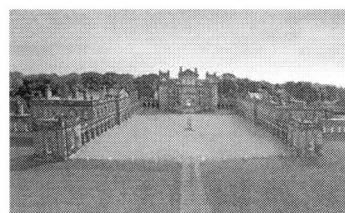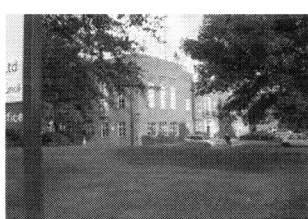

As mentioned earlier I had to find myself a part time job to keep the wolves from the door and I was unbelievably fortunate to be offered the position of Millennium funding officer for the Borough of Blyth Valley. My boss was a wonderful guy called Chris Simpson whose favourite line after every team meeting was "Mek a difference", what a great line which I still use today (check my LinkedIn page). Basically, when you go to work make sure you do one thing that will make a positive difference to either your colleague or the community you serve. If you have a spare five minutes, google Seattle Fish market in the states and you will see something called the Fish Philosophy (read the book). They have put a lot of so called blue chip companies to shame with the way they get through the working day. Make their day, be there and Choose your attitude are the three main principals which dictates their work culture. The thing is, a divvunt think it il catch on doon the Fish Quay.

Anyway, back to Blyth Valley. My role was to get as much funding as possible for community organisations in the Blyth Valley area to celebrate the Millennium. I was employed late 1998 and I had a year or so to work with community groups and associations to develop and deliver as many projects as possible for the new Millennium, and if I say so myself I was pretty successful at it. My target was £50k which I reached after a few of months, by the time I left in 2000 I had pulled in three or four times that amount and I couldn't have helped a better bunch of people.

Northumbrian people in general are honest, hardworking people who are proud of their heritage and the people of Blyth Valley were no different. The area is known for its mining and shipbuilding communities but has now got neither, a bit like my home town of Wallsend, and like Wallsend it had very similar social and economic problems, unemployment and drug misuse to name two. I was fortunate to meet a load of people from a range of community and voluntary organisations who were all giving their time to creating a better place for people to live and at the same time educating people on the heritage of the area and benefits of living in Blyth Valley. I have to say that the culture of Blyth Valley Council in comparison to North Tyneside was poles apart. Staff are an integral part of the system and valued as such. The politics were straight forward to deal with and the councillors were a lot more focussed on collaborating for the betterment of the area rather than trying to score political points whenever the opportunity arose. I'm not saying it was perfect just less politically focussed. Out of all the places I had worked I have never come across the most honest, loyal, helpful and straight-talking people than I did in Blyth Valley and I was genuinely gutted when I left. My colleagues, including the senior management team and the people were an absolute pleasure to work with and what better back drop than the sea to the east and the countryside to the north, all within a five/ten-minute drive. I was offered a permanent contract at Blyth Valley and working for a wonderful guy like Chris Simpson and a team of like-minded people, the offer was tempting but I was desperate to try my hand at the private sector and when the opportunity arose I knew I had to go for it. Thanks for the wonderful experience I had at Blyth Valley and I do hope I did "Mek a difference".

"In the words of my wonderful mam, it's nice to be nice"

Chapter 12

"Baaah its cad" Keeping people warm with Scottish Power

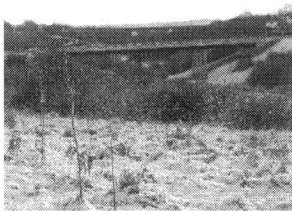

As mentioned above the opportunity I was offered in the private sector came from a subsidiary of Scottish Power from a newly formed company called N.E.S.T.makers. What the job basically entailed was providing free grants to anyone who qualified for draught proofing, loft insulation, cavity wall insulation and central heating. I went through four interviews to get the post and I was really chuffed when I was offered the job as Energy officer?? And asked to attend two weeks of training in Liverpool with colleagues from all over the UK. I was one of eight people who travelled to Liverpool from the North East of England to attend the training and over that period we got to know each other reasonably well as we were living in each other's pockets for two weeks and I have got to say the guys I was going to work with were a canny bunch of mukkas (friends). So, of I trekked to Liverpool with a heavy heart as I was leaving Debbie and the lads for a couple of weeks, I am a deep rooted little bugga who loves travelling but not without my family. Could I work away?? Could I shite.

Once the training was complete I started the job proper which was basically finding customers to offer free energy saving grants and advice, what they failed to tell us at the training was you needed eight appointments a day and you had to offer customers a comparison with their current supplier re gas and electric and then try and get the customer to change to Scottish Power. I really didn't want to do a sales job and I felt I had been hoodwinked by the company on this aspect, but the rest of the job was great, after all I was going to make a lot of people happy and in the bargain, warmer, and reduce their bills. I was also given a spanking brand-new company car, Toyota Yaris verso in racing green, sounds good eh. The lads hated it as it looked a little bit like a posh hearse, they soon came to enjoy the trappings of a new car when I told them to walk to school and we will get the bus to footy training. "Nah, nah yu alright dad we were just joking". Actually, it did look like a posh hearse. The company also provided me with fax, landline and mobile phone, wey man a felt geet posh like.

The job itself was canny. The first week was a bit traumatic; in fact I didn't really have a clue what I was deeying. We all met at our regional office in Gateshead and we were assigned areas, mine being Newcastle, Northumberland and North Tyneside, happy days, I've worked in all those areas. We were then given a weeks' worth of customer contacts and sent on our way with a warning, and it was a warning. "You lot are all on probation so make sure you deliver", in other words if you don't perform yu oot the door bonny lads and lasses. This warning came from our regional manager who to put it bluntly was a "prick" who ruled with fear and focussed his shit "I'm the boss" attitude on the most vulnerable. Now I'm all up for working hard and delivering objectives but people like this guy just wind me up and I turn into a very different character. I basically want to challenge them; nose to nose when the opportunity arises, and it didn't take long before it happened which I will come back to. Anyway, I knew I was going to be alright with my referrals as I had a lot of contacts in the areas I was assigned so of I went on my jolly way. The job seemed like a cross of community development work and sales, the latter being the bit I hated doing. I'm a great pitcher and I can talk passionately about a subject I feel strongly about, for instance offering people the chance to insulate their house but trying to change their energy supplier, well, that just didn't appeal to me at all. It felt a little bit like "I'll give you this, free, if you sign the dotted line for a new energy supplier, although they were under no obligation to switch suppliers and they still got their grant if they qualified. Anyway, crikey I go off on a tangent easily. I survived the first week without too much stress even though my appointments were taking a good hour to carry out and then back home to do the paperwork and then sort appointments out for the next day. I worked twelve/fourteen hour shifts for the first two to three weeks before I really got the hang of the process. By the fourth week I had appointments down to fifteen minutes and I was back home doing my paperwork by 2pm. It was great because I could drop the lads of at school and pick them up which I loved doing.

I had also created a large customer base as I contacted my old colleagues in the areas I was assigned, and I went and done presentations to a whole range of voluntary groups re the grant scheme, this generated a huge amount of appointments which I shared with some of my NESTmaker colleagues who were struggling for appointments. After the first month, we were given our sales figures which I was more than happy with. The prick of a boss I mentioned earlier absolutely berated some of the other staff for not reaching their targets, he had some staff in tears and then asked for the keys to the company car from one guy and when the guy asked him why, he give him a smug grin and said "yu sacked, get any personal belongings and get out". I couldn't believe what I was hearing, I was fuckin furious, and I had to say something. "There is a time and a place to do that and it isn't in front of us lot, if that's yu management style then I can't see me staying here much longer". He glared at me and said, "there's the door" pointing to the entrance to the office. I backed off and shut me gob, thinking to myself that I needed this job.

It became abundantly clear that we were going to be managed by fear rather than by encouragement and support, welcome to the private sector!!!!, no one could run to their union rep crying grievance, it was a case of knuckling down and getting the job done until such time where I can kick the legs away from this fuckin bully of a man. It's just not in my nature to act like this until I am provoked and there is no other avenue to take, after all I was brought up on a cooncil estate where you had to look after yourself and my mam and dad taught us all to defend our corner whenever we felt we were being threatened and this was one such time. I decided to keep a log of his bullying and after meeting the rest of my colleagues away from the office it was decided that we needed to support each other to get through these issues together. To cut a very long and laborious story short I became the designated spokesperson for the group and after another month of threats and bollickings, even though the guys were delivering above expectation I took matters into my own hands and, without speaking to any of my colleagues as I didn't want to put them at risk I rang the HR director and informed him of the problems and the aggressive management style of this numpty. I knew it was a dangerous move because there was a good chance of me being kicked out the organisation, but this guy was absolutely horrified to hear of the things

that were going on and two days later I was summoned to a hotel in Newcastle to meet the chief executive, I was shitting myself and was confident that this would be my last day in the job.

The chief executive listened to everything I had to say and then thanked me for meeting him. He then said "Wally, why have you put yourself at risk basically telling me what you have just told me", my response was "because it's wrong and no person, regardless of their position should be treated in the way some of your staff are being treated and if you feel I am in the wrong then there is no need to sack me, I quit". "You're not being sacked, and you don't have to leave, this will be sorted once I look into it further". Two days later we were all summoned to head office and introduced to our new regional manager and informed that the numpty had been moved elsewhere. I was gobsmacked but delighted that this company did value its staff and the work they were doing. If we were all sitting on our arses and just whining about nowt, then I wouldn't have been surprised to be sacked but we were all grafting like hell to make this company a success and the hierarchy recognised this. The assumption by a lot of people is that the private sector is a more volatile and unpredictable place to work, and I agree with this, after all, if there not making money, then they are out of business and it is your employees who will make the money for you, so they are a priceless asset for your organisation. The private sector (in most organisations) rewards staff for hard work and delivering the outputs in a much better way than the public sector. The public sector has a mental safety net that we will be pulled out the crap by someone in government.

"A solid organisational structure and an engaged workforce are the foundations of success"

How many times in the public sector have you seen people under perform on their targets and still be rewarded with a pay rise in another expensive and irrational restructure or just moved elsewhere, and I say this with experience as it has happened to me, its crazy man? I am not suggesting we sack everyone who we think is shite at their job, bloody hell if we did that we would have next to no politicians!!, I'm saying we shouldn't reward failure or underachievement with promotions or otherwise, we should support these people through training and development. We put to many people in posts they are not capable of doing because they have neither the experience nor knowledge to do this. It happens a lot less now than it used to but it still does happen.

I did have one absolutely bizarre incident happen to me when working for N.E.S.T.makers. I had booked in most of my appointments in the Newcastle area for this day and headed up there after I had dropped the lads off at school. I got through the morning really quickly and I had two more appointments which I had kept until last as I knew they were for central heating systems, which take a bit longer.

Anyway, I knocked on this guy's door a couple of times and there was no answer, so I went back to the car and rang his mobile which he answered. I informed him that I was contacting him re the appointment he had made for the grant and if he was unavailable can we make a new appointment, he said "im in the fuckin hoos man, yu mustn't have knocked hard enough, al get the door". He opened the front door and he filled the whole frame, he was about 6ft5" and built like a brick shithouse wearing a geet big terry towelling dressing gown. I entered the house behind him and immediately felt uncomfortable, there were no carpets throughout the flat and the only furniture on show was one single chair in the living room and an old t.v. set and he seemed angry for some reason. "av been graftin al neet so am knackad, al a want is me fuckin central heating man and a betta get it mind or al fuckin kick off", I was shitting myself and I genuinely felt threatened by this fella. I started to look for something to clout him with if he came for me but there was nowt, the only thing I had was me fuckin clip board and I divvunt think that was gannin to stop him. I went through the form and it was blatantly obvious that he DID NOT qualify for anything other than getting his doors draught proofed but there was no way I was telling him that, he would have kicked the shite out of me. Anyway, I went through the form and he kept saying "do a qualify, do a fucking qualify or wot man", "wey I yu qualify yu gan a get the whole wack", I was lying through *me* teeth, but it was the only way to pacify him. He seemed to calm down and sat on this one chair, and as he sat his arse down on the chair his dressing gown opened revealing his bloody meat and two veg. "Oh fuck", I said to myself, I need to get out of here quick sharpish. I calmly said to him that I just needed to measure the doors in the passage to make sure he got all his draught proofing, he remained seated as I walked past him, and I quickly made a very quiet and quick exit from his house. I ran like hell towards the car when I heard him shouting from his living room "hoy where the fuck are yu goin", I started the car and wheel spinned out of his street. He was running behind me shouting and screaming with his dressing gown wide open and everything dangling and swinging. I didn't stop driving until I pulled into my drive and then breathed a huge sigh of relief. I rang the office and explained everything and said I was doing nee more appointments today. It was one of the scariest and traumatic things I have went through.   When I reflect on this story I think of those people who do this day in, day out in my current organisation, particularly district nurses, health visitors, mental health workers, GPs and all those other workers who undertake lone working and who put themselves at risk every single day of the week when trying to deliver a safe and efficient service for patients. Not long after that incident I decided it was time to move on even though I was enjoying my job I was becoming bored with doing the same thing day in day out and the most important aspect of my working life is supporting and working alongside colleagues, so finding myself on the road each day running from house to house, estate to estate had become rather tedious and boring. I was paid well, had a company car and a very rewarding job but there were no challenges for me to get my teeth into, so I decided I would look for something which was more focused on, community development work or the likes.

"If you think the world owes you something then think again, or you will never succeed in anything"

Chapter 13

Life in the NHS

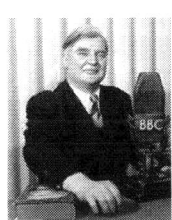

"The NHS will last as long as there are folk left with faith to fight for it" —*AneurinBevan*

Make sure you are one of those people. We have the best health system in the world, free at the point of entry and we need to keep it that way.

I stumbled into the NHS rather than chose this as a career, but it has become a passion and an ambition to provide the best service possible to the people of North Tyneside and across the NHS system, that's not bullshit, it's a fact. As already mentioned I was looking for something more challenging when I came across an advert for a Healthy community's worker for the North Tyneside area, I couldn't believe my luck. I applied and got the job on a one-year contract which suited me perfectly as at the time I was quite happy jumping from job to job, well fourteen years later and I am still there albeit in another role from when I started but still in the NHS.

The NHS is a strange beast and it took me a while to feel comfortable in its culture which varies from team to team, department to department and organisation to organisation. In comparison (at the time I started in 2001) to the local authority the NHS had a less aggressive culture to it and it was much more academically focused and a lot less political which surprised me as I assumed that these people would have been much more politically astute but that wasn't the case. I am still surprised that this theme (one of the only ones remaining) has continued to this day. We all know how the NHS has become a political football, but staff still seem quite oblivious to this and I don't think we use this to our advantage. Anyway, I will get into this issue later on, for now I am going to give you a breakdown of my roles within the NHS over the past fourteen years and then talk about some of the pitfalls, hurdles and accomplishments of that work and in doing so I hope to highlight some of the wonderful teams and individuals I have had the privilege of working with and also some of the bullshitters, power trippers and snobs I have had the unfortunate pleasure of coming across.

The following is a list of jobs I have had and the organisations I have worked for and on only one occasion did I move by choice, the rest of my moves were through re-organisation and national strategic changes or goal post moving, whichever you prefer.

- Healthy Communities worker – Health Action Zone/Healthy community's programme
- Healthy Community's worker – North Tyneside PCT
- Healthy Living Centre Manager – North Tyneside PCT
- Head of community Health Development – North Tyneside PCT
- Primis worker – North Tyneside PCT
- Operational Manager – North Tyneside PCT
- Transformation officer – Newcastle and North Tyneside Community Health
- Operational Estates Manager – Newcastle and North Tyneside community Health (secondment)
- Transformation Officer – Newcastle and North Tyneside Community Health
- Transformation Lead – Northumbria Healthcare Hospital Trust

- Head of Transformation and Change – North Tyneside Clinical Commissioning Group

PHEWWW I had forgot how many jobs I have done, and I have learnt and developed immensely from the experiences. Within that period of time I have went through six re-organisations with three of them being centrally implemented (government) and the rest being knock on effects from those changes and here is the irony. I am sitting in my current role in a building I was based in and a desk I occupied seven years ago with a different role and organisation, you tell me if that is a good use of public money???? I think not. What I think is that it was politically motivated following an ideological strategy of the current government. Some benefits but some absolutely irrational political strategies that cost the tax payer a fortune and created low morale and confusion across the health care system. What I do think is that the current Health Secretary has created a steady pair of hands (Didn't think I would here myself saying that) but is still dismantling the NHS in his own quiet way, after his incompetent numpty of a colleague was moved sideways. Another public servant rewarded for failure.

Anyway, back to the more interesting stuff (I think!!!), life in the NHS has been a roller coaster of a ride and in the main a really enjoyable ride. I have had the good fortune to support the real heroes of the NHS, Nurses, doctors, Health visitors, District nurses and all the other clinicians who do a phenomenal job saving lives and caring for people. Until you have lived it and breathed it you will not appreciate their commitment, passion and compassion. In all my roles, I have been the bloke, with a huge amount of other dedicated back office staff who have supported them. If I was to use an analogy, I have always seen my role as a stage hand with the clinicians and front-line staff the actors and stars of the NHS show.

I agree that there have been too many middle management structures which have slowed the system down rather than speeding the system up but this has now dissipated in most cases, but I still think there are too many structural bloody bureaucrats that are employed to stop us delivering rather

71

than supporting us to deliver and these days there is far too much political interference within the system. Make absolutely no doubts about it; the NHS is hierarchical both clinically and academically. I struggled trying to understand the concept when I first joined as I see everyone as equal but the difference I found in the NHS in comparison with the local authority (the council) was this attitude of superiority. I have got to say, that fourteen years on and this attitude still remains in large parts of the NHS which is absolutely shameful. Old fashioned management styles and an unwillingness to change has cut across all the different areas of the NHS but the paradox is there are more staff who are embracing change for the betterment of the patients that use their services. Some of this is forced through political involvement and government targets and some of it has just happened through innovative and strong leadership.

Some of that innovation and leadership was evident in my first role where we developed a Healthy Communities Programme where voluntary groups from the local community could apply for funding up to £5k to develop a local health project which focused on community involvement and engagement and obviously, health benefits. Representatives from the organisations were also panel members on the funding group that awarded the grants. My role was to work with the panel members and then to support the groups who were funded to help them develop their project. This was putting the decisions into the hands of the volunteers who knew their community better than any professional, but they were supported by those professionals on a number of occasions to add value to the projects. We had parent and toddler, knit and natter, schools, football clubs, photography groups, youth groups and a load more of community organisations. One of the most successful outcomes for me was the funding and development of the VINE which is now a little community café in Howdon. It was originally a bank which was converted in to the community drop in and when we talk about leaders there was none better than Reverend Joan Dotchin. Now I'm not a religious bloke, in fact the total opposite but when we talk about people who inspire others, Joan was one of those people and as stupid as it sounds, I never seen her as a reverend I only seen her as a person to rely on.

I was based in the VINE for a short period of time, upstairs in one of the offices so I had the good fortune to regularly chat to the good folk of Howdon that came in for a cuppa and a knatta and browsed through the clothes and the books which were sold. On one such occasion I was chatting to a young mother who always came into the VINE after she had dropped her two young bairns off at school. They were about seven and five years old. It was obvious, and she made it clear in conversation that she didn't have two pennies to rub together but she wanted the best for her kids and she always bought those bairns something, either clothes, books or on the odd occasion some kets (sweets). I knew then that the VINE was going to be a success and since that day many more local people have popped into the VINE for a chat and cuppa. I haven't got any statistical analysis to back up what I am saying but I do have a huge amount of empirical evidence which tells me that there were both health and social benefits attached to that project.

Some people have many names for community groups and activists, some good some bad, but communities would be a much less vibrant place without them. They give their time free and provide a number of services for young and old which would otherwise not be available. I can count on one hand the "bad uns", the cliques and the "do gooders" and I can offer a hundred plus "good uns" from Blyth to wallsend and Walker to Wheatslade. If you are a so called professional whether a nurse, health visitor or community worker expect conflict when you are working with these people but say nowt and listen to what they have to say. Don't respond with corporate bullshit or patronising crap. Respond with a positive, and a solution but let them know that they will need to work with you to get a positive outcome. I have a principal I always work to with all people be that community reps or staff and its:

"Include people and they will respond, exclude people and they will react".

Over the next twelve years of my life in the NHS I undertook a lot of roles and experienced some wonderful and inspirational pieces of work, but I have also experienced some crap, well haven't we all. So, let me explain a bit more about that last sentence and let's start with the good stuff.

I have worked for five different organisations in my fourteen years in the NHS which says a lot about the ever-changing organisational restructure and reform programmes the bloody politicians feel need to happen. As already mentioned my work in Healthy communities delivered a number of projects across the whole health spectrum and one of those projects was carried forward into North Tyneside PCT. That project was, for me one of the most successful projects ever to come out of North Tyneside and it was the Healthy Living centres. Originally a funded scheme through the Big Lottery Fund and then mainstreamed by the PCT.

"Unity is a signal of hope and can't be ignored"

The project was managed by a group of local people and health staff and it is safe to say that it was unbelievably difficult to get agreement on the structure of the HLCs and what criteria was going to be put in place. My role in this project was to manage it as I was now Head of Community Health development and as you will read later it nearly sent me to an early grave. The funding for this project would never have been achieved if it was not for the voluntary groups and there representatives being active partners in the scheme but creating an open access service was so difficult as these groups all wanted a major piece of the pie for their groups, which is understandable and in my way of thinking correct but how some of these people conducted themselves was unreasonable and in some cases just personalised egotism which had no place in what we were trying to achieve. As mentioned earlier you will have conflict but this wasn't conflict it was just uncalled-for manipulation which, to cut a long story short was resolved when the funding ended and the PCT took on the management of the programme.

Now, community activists are absolute gold dust and I am passionate about supporting their ideas, issues and concerns but if you are a community activist you have a responsibility to your community and everyone in that community and not just the chosen few which on this occasion, in some quarters but not all, was the case.
Once all the politics and power trips were resolved the HLCs went from strength to strength providing an unbelievable service for the people of North Tyneside and the person who drove the success of the HLCs was a woman called Maureen Turner, who is one of the most loyal, passionate and knowledgeable individuals I have had the pleasure of working with. She engaged with volunteers, patients, users, acute trusts, universities, consultants, GPs, social clubs and even bingo organisations to get her message across re the service the HLCs provided and there was no one who

knew that service better than Maureen. The staff within the HLCs were just as committed as Maureen and were unbelievably qualified in the work they delivered. People need to understand the commitment of these staff. This may have been a job they were paid to do but they went way past their pay grade and they had an excellent relationship with the users of the HLCs. Two of the best projects ever to come out of North Tyneside are "Into Work"

and the Healthy Living Centres, don't take my word for it just ask the thousands of people who have accessed these services and the mental, social and health benefits they have delivered for those users. Unfortunately, both services have now been cut for financial and strategic reasons!!!!! My arse.

I have, and always will class myself as an NHS worker as long as I am in post. I am currently working in a CCG (I've gone to the dark side) where we commission services to other NHS organisations, Local Authorities and also private and third sector companies and organisations but I see them as colleagues and not bloody enemies or threats, but how the system is set up, finance and performance rule the roost (obviously) which creates animosity and a lot of negotiating and bickering re who gets what. In other words, we have created an internal market which has little benefit for patients as we are all trying to either make a buck and more, or commission services on very low margins. My solution, and pardon me for being so dumb, but stick it all in the same pot or using government speak, create an integrated care solution. No shit Sherlock. In the words of Richard Branson (Founder of Virgin) "complexity is your enemy. Any fool can make something complicated. It is hard to make something simple".
The NHS is one complex mess of organisations (fifth largest employer in the world, 1.7 million). Now as a patient, the vast majority of people see it as all one organisation and rightly so, but as a worker, well, it's a bloody nightmare to put it bluntly and so frustrating. I am sure the NHS have complexity managers but under a different name as they come up with some weird and wonderful strategies and organisational structures. The people who suffer because of this complexity are the patients and the front-line staff dealing with them.

I find it quite humorous that we spend more time looking at other health systems, the Americans and the Swedes to name but two when actually we are ranked higher than both as published by THE Guardian on Tuesday 17th June 2014 by Denis Campbell and Nicholas Watt this is also supported by the World Health Organisation.

"No system survives unless we collaborate to succeed"

I do think it is important to look at what other people are doing but we then need to look at what we need to do to improve the current system, but we seem to jump on the band wagon of introducing this from that country and that from another when actually we just need to have some stability in our own system with minimal changes unless necessary. The trouble is it all costs money and we haven't got enough so we cut, cut, cut or make "efficiency plans", one of the same to me. All this does is create an opportunity for some smart arse in Whitehall to write another national strategy or reform programme which has little or no comparison to the real world but is built on financial data and modelling. The bottom line is we need investment in the system and if we want to continue to have a NHS which is free to the UK population then it will need to be paid for centrally. If we haven't got the money, then stop piss farting about with inefficient change models and privatise the whole system and then let's see the kick back that creates!!!

Let's take an example of political reform.

Perhaps most infamously, the Conservatives repeatedly promised before the general election (2010) that there would be no more "top-down re-organisations" of the NHS (*Andrew Lansley, Conservative Party press release, 11 July 2007*). In a speech at the Royal College of Pathologists on 2 November 2009, Cameron said: "With the Conservatives there will be no more of the tiresome, meddlesome, top-down re-structures that have dominated the last decade of the NHS." http://www.newstatesman.com/politics/2013/11/pre-election-pledges-tories-are-trying-wipe

Then post 2010 election we endured the most radical and largest reform programme in the NHS history which has created continued turmoil for all sectors of the NHS and created a huge amount of stress and uncertainty for staff. The basis of the change was under the guise of austerity and efficiency, but the reality of the situation was confusion, uncertainty and unnecessary change. More restructuring and more accountability, creating more beaurocracy and tiers of structure. I am aware that people got substantial pensions (nowhere near as big as banker's bonuses by the way) but they didn't set the rules and they certainly didn't enter the NHS thinking "ill forge a career with the NHS because the pension scheme is great". I have read and listened to so many people with a view on this, that, like a lot of people, I just shrug my shoulders apathetically and switch off.

While I am on me rant I just want to put something to bed. I have no issue with the private sector and the people who work in it so why has this government targeted public sector workers as being the people who have created the current financial mess we are in and haled the private sector as the saviours for the future. Like most people I fell into my work and I have worked in both sectors and believe me, one will not work without the other so stop all this bullshit and focus on reality. In my opinion the NHS is doomed as long as it is used as a political football between numpty politicians and as long as we keep developing systems for reporting rather than systems for patients. I am bored shitless attending meetings with a focus on KPIs, outcomes, trajectories and return on investments instead of listening to real patient stories and frontline staff ideas to implement real change and improve care, cost and experience.

To finish on this rather tedious and emotive rant I want to tell you about my current experience. I am one of many staff who are currently working in an organisation who are in financial recovery, wu skint in other words. Every Wednesday our director team gather around a telephone to have the shit kicked out of them by NHS officials who focus on finance and outcomes and bloody theoretical fuckin action plans, they just want the books to balance. Well im afraid yu bunch of egotistic, we know best, paper pushing numpties are wrong and you are picking on the wrong people. Do your homework and look at the unbelievably well performing trusts that we commission and then look at failing trusts in other areas, guess what their CCGs are cash rich. Are you seeing the pattern, its similar across the country? If you want quality services you have to pay for them or you can always bend the rules and falsify the figures, like Mid Staffs, which would you prefer?? The system is broken and unless there is investment it will disappear like the sunset but fail to rise. RANT OVER, well nearly.

The NHS has changed in form, shape, size and principal and will never return to pre-2010 structures. It is more complex now than it has ever been, and things will get worse. The system is now dictated by smart arse eye watering over paid consultants, analysts and financial experts who would not recognise a patient if they were slapped in the face by them. Doctors, nurses and other frontline staff have very little control. GPs are making decisions on rules dictated to them by CCGs which are based on finance and not patient experience. Like I have said before, if we want a first-class service then we will have to pay for it or, if this current government has its way we can create a health class system which will involve either paying direct or paying through insurance or in the worst case just doing some DIY healthcare for those who can't afford it. Take a long hard look at the failing American system, do we really want that health system. This report headline was from Michael Hiltzik (The Economy Hub, June 17th 2014). **The U.S. healthcare system ranks last among 11 developed countries, according to a new study by the Commonwealth Fund. (Commonwealth Fund)** Is this the future, I hope not, or we are totally fucked.

I have held many posts in the NHS and worked with god knows how many people. One thing is for sure, the vast majority of those people are absolutely dedicated to delivering a fantastic service to the people of the United Kingdom. They are unsung heroes who regularly work way over their hours and as for seven day working, well no shit Sherlock, of course this should happen but unless the Health Secretary is going to knit some GPs or magic some nurses it will never get off the ground. It is all aspirational rhetoric with no real commitment to implementation.

I am not scare mongering I am being absolutely serious, we are in a very, very dark place at the moment and unless people wake up to the fact that this current governments ideology is just so unfair then we will lose our fantastic and world-famous health service.

> "Illness is neither an indulgence for which people have to pay, nor an offence for which they should be penalised, but a misfortune, the cost of which should be shared by the community."
>
> Aneurin Bevan - founder of the NHS

"Patients and frontline staff need to be listened to and we need to stop counting widgets for the sake of politicians"

Chapter 14

Organisational Culture

I will end this section repeating part of my introduction. I have had an interesting work journey where I have experienced a whole range of cultures, good, bad and fuckin awful but one thing has remained the same and it is change, it is inevitable which then dictates culture and behaviour, you then end up with the following:

- The rebels and reformists
- The different classes/hierarchies
- The autocratic and the engagers,
- Academics and the experienced
- the politics and the power trips
- the deceit and the delight,
- the bullshit and the rhetoric,
- the passionate and the innovators,
- the creative and the bureaucrats,
- the shirkers and the workers,
- the compassionate and the bullies,
- the front-line staff and the management,
- the theorists and the pragmatists,
- the doers and the do nothings,
- the jokers and the jesters,

- the leaders and the followers,
- the wingers and the moaners,
- the inspirers and the inspired,

Dealing with some of these people above is either a pain in the arse or a pleasure and I have experienced all of them. The question is, would an organisation suffer or survive if some of these people weren't there. My work life would have been pretty boring if I didn't have the pleasure of crossing paths with these people and I would have not been able to develop half the interpersonal and engagement skills I have.

To conclude I would say that from the shipyards to present day I have experienced a whole variation of cultures but all with common themes which has been a variation of the above. No matter where you work and no matter what decade you have worked in you will experience good people, irrational people, power people, egotistic people, bullies and bullshitters, story tellers and risk takers. You will have opportunity doors opened and then the same doors slammed in your face. You will have flexible working and rigid shift patterns and you will always moan about management and salaries and then become one of them yourself. Technology continues to evolve and forge ahead but don't over complicate the fact that we have never really changed. Fashion, technology, equality and travel has changed beyond recognition, but the culture of organisations has not shifted and I very much doubt that it will. People are people and regardless of what I am told or what I read I know that you will always come across that bulleted list I mentioned at the start of this chapter. Christ, if all people were hard working, never sick and as good as gold then we could get rid of human resources and occupational health. But we haven't got that anywhere in any organisation. What effects how employees operate and work, is the hierarchy. If you treat people like shite and pay them coppers, you tend to get a workforce that are pissed off with little commitment. If you treat your workforce with respect, provide a good working environment then you usually get a loyal and committed staff, yes, some people take the piss but in the main people do what they are paid to do and more.

I am no organisational guru I am just speaking from experience. I will leave the theory to the academics and researchers, I am just telling you what I have seen, heard and tasted over the past thirty-six years.

Let's not fool ourselves, we are who we are and there is good, bad, fluffy and funny thinking people we work with and whether you work in retail, technology, engineering, health or anywhere else you will know who these people are, and long may it continue, they form organisational culture, they make it come alive. The only thing I would want to change is the fucking "meeting" bullshitters, those people who spend their working lives attending meetings, saying the same thing and delivering absolutely nowt or presenting a paper which goes nowhere, get rid of them they are a waste of space, time, energy and money.

My working life has been a funny old journey and I have done jobs because I needed to work or nee bugga could have paid the bills. I have emptied the copper jar to pay for the bairns dinner money and I have took oot Provi loans to make sure the bairns got what they wanted for Christmas and I am unashamedly proud of the fact that I now don't have to do that and I can, to a certain extent choose where I wish to live, work and purchase most things I want for me or the family. I have learnt how to deal with a whole range of personal issues and people because of those jobs I have done. One thing is for certain I owe those people a lot as they inadvertently have taught me to respect people and never, ever change who you are because of your position because some smart arse fucka will shoot you down. I can categorically say that my principals and ethics have remained the same throughout my career and I will never shift from that position. I respect people because of their patta and personality not their position or power and long may that continue. I have endured stress related illness which has left its scars or in the words of my wonderful GP "MY GREMLINS", but I have learnt to accept them and deal with them. I have learnt how to manage stress and pressure and I know when to challenge or contribute so thanks to everyone I have worked with, good, bad or plain arrogant arse holes, you have all taught me a lot.

"Life is one long strange journey, deal with the downs, celebrate the ups, strive to be a better person"

Chapter 15

The Working-Class Syndrome

"This business of petty inconvenience and indignity, of being kept waiting about, of having to do everything at other people's convenience, is inherent in working-class life. A thousand influences constantly press a working man down into a passive role. He does not act; he is acted upon. He feels himself the slave of mysterious authority and has a firm conviction that 'they' will never allow him to do this, that, and the other. Once when I was hop-picking I asked the sweated pickers (they earn something under sixpence an hour) why they did not form a union. I was told immediately that 'they' would never allow it. Who were 'they'? I asked. Nobody seemed to know, but evidently 'they' were omnipotent." George Orwell, The Road to Wigan Pier

That is the working-class syndrome.

Agree or disagree, I really couldn't give a shite, but the working-class syndrome exists, even today. We are told from an early age that we will aspire to this or we won't aspire to that and because of the historical past of our family's work and educational attainment we usually set our sights to low and we are told not to get "too big for our boots". The principal goes back generations and is instilled in the vast majority of working class families. This is forced upon us from a very early age and a lot of it depends on where we live. Please don't think that I am having a pop at people who have not experienced the syndrome because I'm not. This is definitely less apparent

82

today but if you are raised on a council estate or an area of deprivation you will usually have to deal with all the shit that goes with that. More crime, fewer amenities, drug abuse, ante social behaviour and stigma, and with stigma comes assumptions. Assumptions by your family, teachers, law enforcement, the council and health authorities and bloody politicians, and to try and get out of that circle is difficult but not impossible.

It's hard to put my finger on the problem but to back up my theory the people who run our country are all from wealthy privately educated families who have this fucking irritating thing of rolling up their sleeves when they are going to do a bit graft.

They tell us we are "in it together" or that they're not afraid of making the tough decisions. There's nowt tough about cutting people's disability allowance or sticking room tax on some pensioners three bedroomed house that he/she has lived in for fifty years, that's not tough that's cowardly and unethical. So why do they do it??? They have no understanding, concept or feeling towards people from these areas but they know that they really don't want them to develop into an educated and confident individual who may challenge their principals, assumptions and ideology.

What section of the above picture do you fit into and more importantly what section did your parents/grandparents fit into. I think this is an excellent image which shows the people who generate the wealth for the few who benefit from the hard work and struggles of the working class.

What I am trying to say in this section of my ramblings is that if you want it, go and get it, legally. Work hard, study like hell and get a qualification or a good trade but for god's sake don't expect any help from the powers that be because they see you as a threat. If you accept that you will never make anything of your life then bigger fool you, they have beat you down to a point of submission where you are happy to sit on your arse and be told what you can and can't have or do. Fight back, prove people wrong, focus on a person who said you would never be anything and prove them wrong. Find your financial

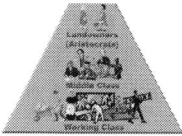

"Over decades we have been told that we should be thankful for what we have, should we really?"

and personal level that you are happy with and then stick two fingers up to those people who thought you would never be that person and tell them "I told you so".

I am proud to be working class and my principals have remained the same although if I was to give my personal details to a poll I would be told I am middle class and I would be comfortable with that statement. I have a good job, a decent hoos and a nice car and I can have a couple of holidays a year and treat my family when I want to. I'm not rich or well off I'm just comfortable, financially and mentally. I'm at the level I wanted to aspire to, so "up yours" to all those people who said I wouldn't do anything with my life.

> And my two wonderful sons support my comment

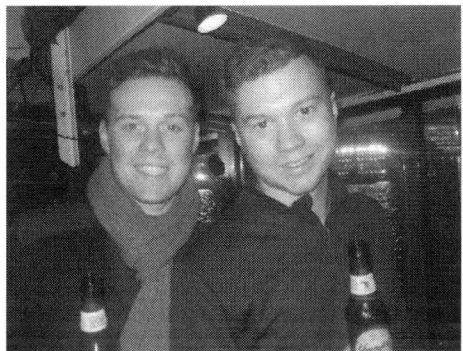

"Don't accept mediocracy, reach for the stars and see where you end up"

Chapter 16

Personal and Professional life – Do they mix?

I would be lying through me teeth if I said they didn't mix, because in most cases you don't have an option, but one thing I make sure I do is pick and choose when I want them to mix and when I don't.

I mentally switch into work mode when I leave my hoos in the morning and I mentally switch off from work when I walk oot the office door on a night time, easier said than done but I do it.

I am a great believer in the theory that your quality of life at work should be the best it can be and that means that you are supported correctly by your employer. You have the right tools to do the job and you are paid a decent salary for what you do. Some people come to work and use it in a positive way as a release from the pressures of home life or the reverse. But the best scenario is a positive balance of both sides which is a lot more difficult to achieve. Usually if you're happy at work then you don't take negative shit home with you which helps to create a happy personal life. Unfortunately, it sometimes doesn't work the other way.

I am fortunate as I love my job and I respect and appreciate my colleagues, but it wasn't always like that. In 2004 I did take my work home to the point where it took over my life, stressed me out to the point of spending five months on the sick. The impact can be devastating so I am writing this short chapter to advise you not to feel frightened to say, "I'm struggling" either personally or professionally. Seek some help before it bites you on the arse and creates a long, long road to recovery. I was fortunate as I had a supportive family and a director who is the most compassionate and hard-working person I have ever come across and now a really good mate, Dr Lesley Young Murphy, who saved my career at that point, as I was ready to "chuck in the towel". Don't stick yu heed in the sand, stand tall and ask for help, you will be amazed how many people want to help you and even more amazed to find out how many of your colleagues have been in a similar position.

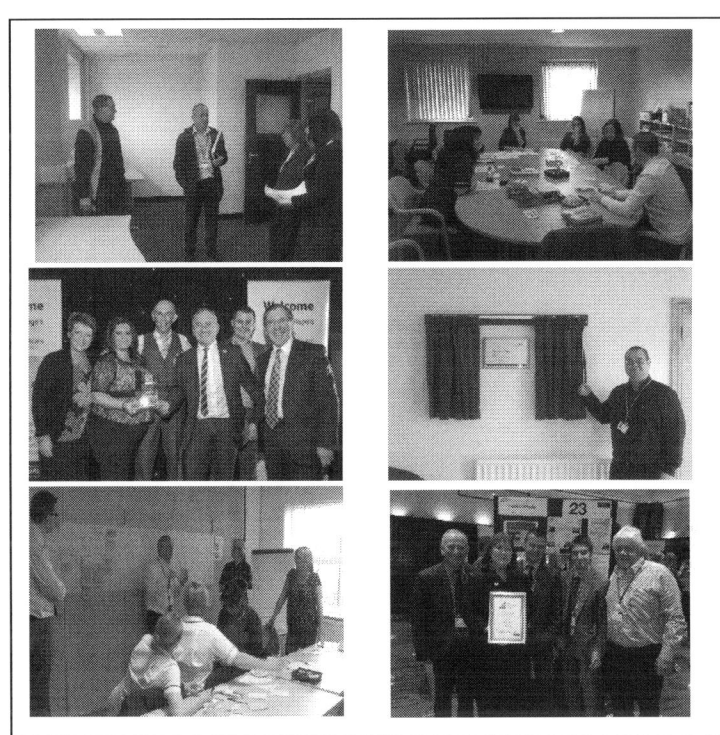

"Stress is an illness so no matter where you sit in the hierarchy seek help when you need it"

Chapter 17
Leaders Mentors and People, I respect

During my working life, I have had the privilege to work with some wonderful, inspirational human beings. Some leaders, some followers and some managers but all have left their mark on the way I work. I have no intention of writing reams of soft centred bullshit about them I'm just going to mention them by name and where appropriate write a line or two about them.

- Tommy Moss
- Tommy Shipley
- Bill Shafto
- Geordie Forest
- Derek Hastings
- Stevie Johnson
- Roy Murphy
- Eddie Barras
- Gladys Wilson – I learnt so much from Gladys through her unassuming way of supporting and guiding you to where you needed to be. Calmness personified.
- Tommy Wilson
- Mala Henderson
- Charlie Scott
- Peter Kirkley
- Jill Prendergast
- Maurya Cushlow – No nonsense, but fair
- Mario Bernardi
- Big Stevie Jackson
- Ashley Charlton
- Margaret Wright
- Mick Tait
- Keeks McGarry
- Chris Simpson – An amazing supportive and inspirational guy
- Alan Davison
- Reverend Joan Dotchin
- Brian Topping
- All North Tyneside District Nurses
- Alex Dougal – Always in the background but a great person to have alongside you
- Sheila Moore
- Maureen Turner
- Michele Spencer
- Kelly Scott
- Ali Corrie
- All the HLC gym staff
- All the volunteers I have had the privilege to work with
- Dr Gbenga Afolobi

- Anne Timmins
- Marc Rice
- Dr Lesley Young Murphy – My mentor, mate and inspiration. She is a leader of people and should be recognised for her unbelievable skill to motivate and generate enthusiasm amongst colleagues and geet clever
- Gary Charlton
- Mal Charlton
- Paul Doohan
- Jade Rainey
- All staff at NTCCG
- Adrian Dracup
- Dr Mark Westwood
- Christine Davison
- Jeff Goldthorpe
- Craig Charlton
- Liam Charlton
- Andrew Charlton
- IT engineers
- Bev Charlton
- Christine Davison

The biggest influence on my working and personal life has been my family, especially my wonderful wife who has stood by me solidly through the good and not so good times. I can honestly say my life would be in ruins if it wasn't for this rock of an individual. I love her loads. I am fortunate to have two wonderful inspirational sons who have made me and Debbie immensely proud of their achievements and their continued drive to be successful, both professionally and personally, they continue to make us unbelievably proud parents and a wonderful daughter in law, Ashleigh and future daughter in law, Lucy who keep me grounded and sane, I love them all dearly and one very special lady who has melted my heart and reinvigorated me and Debbie's life, our beautiful granddaughter, Eleanor Rose who celebrates her first Christmas this year (2015).

So, let me introduce you to my wonderful family in pictures.

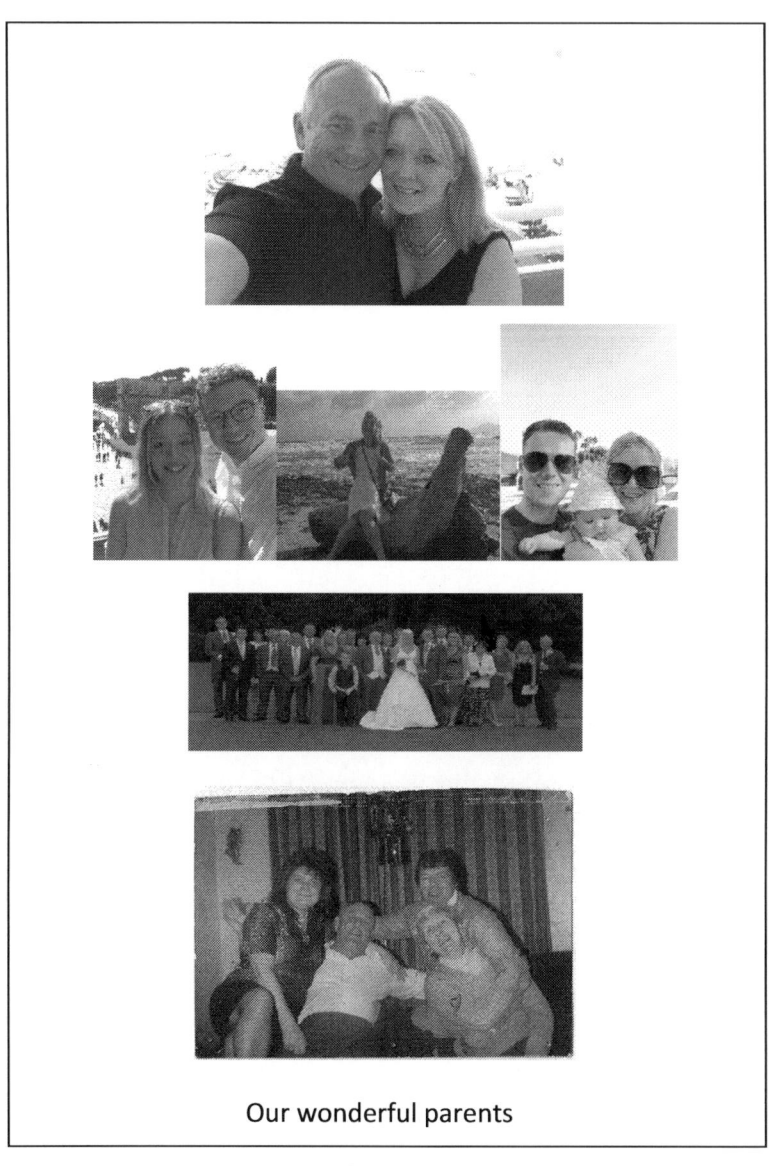

Our wonderful parents

Chapter 18

Academia

I've got to say academia has never been one of my favourite things to do but it wasn't until I left high school that I realised the importance of education. For some reason, although I done ok at school (Eight CSEs and one O, Level) I never enjoyed being taught. This may have had something to do with me not being a conformist or generally treating the whole school thing as a bit of a laugh. It wasn't until I started my apprenticeship that I realised I should have listened and studied a bit more, so I knew I had some catching up to do and this catching up started at the Charles Trevelyan College where we were sent on six-week block placements during the year to learn the theory of engineering and I was gobsmacked that I enjoyed the vast majority of those weeks studying, and I must have been listening because I passed all the exams.

Without boring you about my academic history I have since studied at diploma, national certificate, degree and master degree level and surprised myself and passed all the relevant criteria, it is fair to say that I also shocked a lot of other people. I talk how I talk with a quite broad and localised Geordie accent which I am proud of and won't change for anybody and some people turn their nose up because they have already made an assumption about me which pisses me off no end but I know I can also use it as a tool to trip some smart arse bullshitter up, which I do find amusing, childish you may think and actually I wouldn't disagree but it does show you how some people think they are above others because of the way they talk or where they live, that kind of snobbery just doesn't wash with me.

One of the most rewarding and enjoyable experiences I have had is what I am doing currently. I have, with Marc Rice and Gary Charlton (yes wor Gary, we work for the same organisation) and the continued support and encouragement from Dr Lesley Young Murphy, developed a web based Service Improvement/Project management toolkit called the CQI (Continuous Quality Improvement) which is now being developed into an academic course at levels four to Master's degree. Lesley is a fellow at Northumbria University which has helped to get things started and we are now visiting lecturers (ha-ha, I still find that funny to say) which I am immensely proud of. The course is due to commence sometime next year (2016).

I have learnt so much from studying the theory of a number of subjects and knowing the importance of that theory as I have converged this thinking with the vast amount of practical experience I have developed over the years. The reason I completed my Master's degree was for one reason and one reason only, to prove to myself that I could do it and I wasn't the thick kid from Howdon by the gasworks (back to that working-class syndrome). I was the first person within my immediate family to gain an academic qualification which I'm also very proud of. This doesn't make me any better than anyone else it just means that I was capable of undertaking the task put in front of me and it proves that if I can do this at the ripe old age of fifty years old then anyone can do it regardless of your background and regardless of whether you done well at school or you didn't. The morale of this story is don't be intimidated by people or by your achievements or lack of them. Use this as a motivational tool to get to where you want to be and if you are prepared to listen, study and learn then you will be able to stick yu fingers up at the doubters and piss takers.

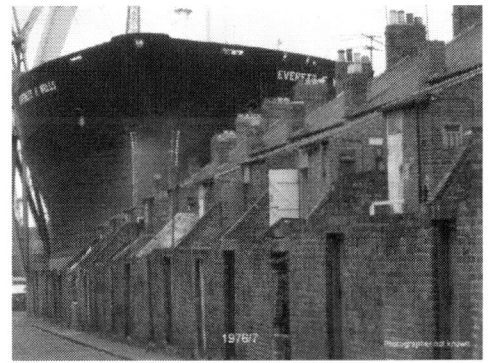

This was the wonderful view I had from my back yard

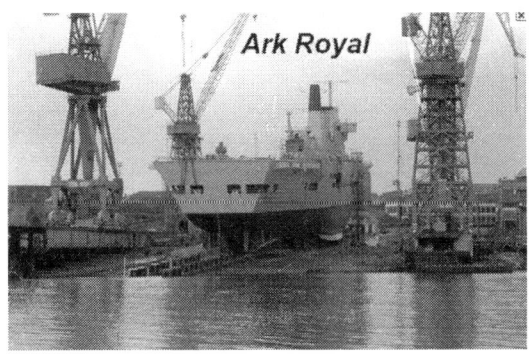

And one of the ships I helped to build, HMS Ark Royal

"Life is a roller coaster but sometimes it feels so good it's like sliding down rainbows"

Chapter 19

Does it matter anyway?

Well of course it matters, it all matters, the laughter, joy, frustration good times and bad because that is life. Agreed, that for some people life is a breeze but no matter who you are we have all got to deal with issues, conundrums, personal and professional problems and decisions. The trick is how you approach it and how you resolve those issues above.

Your working life is, in itself an education. From your first day at work until your last you will be learning new things and dealing with a whole range of issues from accepting orders to dealing with staff and interpersonal relationships and guess what, you'll then go home and use some of those skills you've learnt with yu kids, family members and maraas (mates). If I had my way I would have preferred not to work and just travelled the world, but life, for most of us is not like that so here I am, thirty-six years down the road and still grafting like most people I know.

When I reflect on my working life I tend to focus on what I have achieved and what I have learnt and the characters I have had the pleasure to work with. It's also important to remember the journey I have been on, and what a journey it has been. From that forst day on the 20th August 1979 to present I have been excited, scared, angry, resentful, passive, aggressive, disruptive, brave, innovative, radical and everything else in between and from each one of those feelings I have learnt when and when not to use them both professionally and personally. The first few years were a "right off" because everything I tried to do I got things tits up as you may have read and to this day although I have now learnt to use them wisely I still drop the occasional bollick and sometimes I just do it to either get my point over or shut up a gob shite, but I am still learning. I have grown from a 16-year-old know all to a reasonably calm fifty-two-year-old grandad who has experienced hardship, loss of loved ones, debt, being flush (having a bit money), being married to a beautiful and wonderful wife, and all the joys and stresses that brings, made redundant on more than one occasion, fatherhood, and now I am trying to be a grandad, that's what the point is. Learning to cope and learning to enjoy life as much as possible and feeling fulfilled whether yu minted or skint in work or on the Nat King Coal.

My working life has been a maze, with dead ends, open doors and now I am getting close to the exit door where I will sit back with a pint in my hand and raise my glass to all those people who have helped me get there.

Happy Days.

"Don't be too hard on those who are learning, we've all been there"

Happy Days and thanks

Well, that's it folks, I've rambled through my working life and if you've read this far, well done. I travelled through my working life from a fresh faced 16-year-old to a fifty-two-year-old grandad (doesn't time fly when yu learning). I've tried to give an insight into what I have experienced, learnt and coped with and by doing that I have tried to explain how important culture is in any organisation and I hope you have enjoyed the read and maybe reflected on some of things you have done and some behaviours you have witnessed.

If you want any tips, well, the only one I can give you, is enjoy the highs and deal with the lows and divvunt be a nasty bugga. Treat people with respect and challenge those who don't show any. I've been canny objective in my ramblings and maybe a little bit coy at what I have said as after all I am still grafting. So, in eight years' time I might just do a 2nd edition and say exactly what I want, waarts and al.

Well, am buggaring off now to write some more ramblings, but this time aboot me family life.

Wherever you live, wherever you graft be safe and if all else fails just smile, it always makes yu feel better.

Happy Days

Wally Charlton

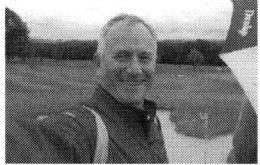

Printed in Great Britain
by Amazon

73123765R00059